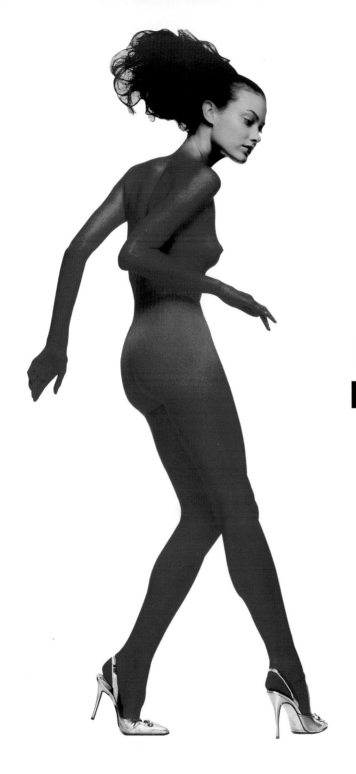

THE
BEAUTY
MANUAL

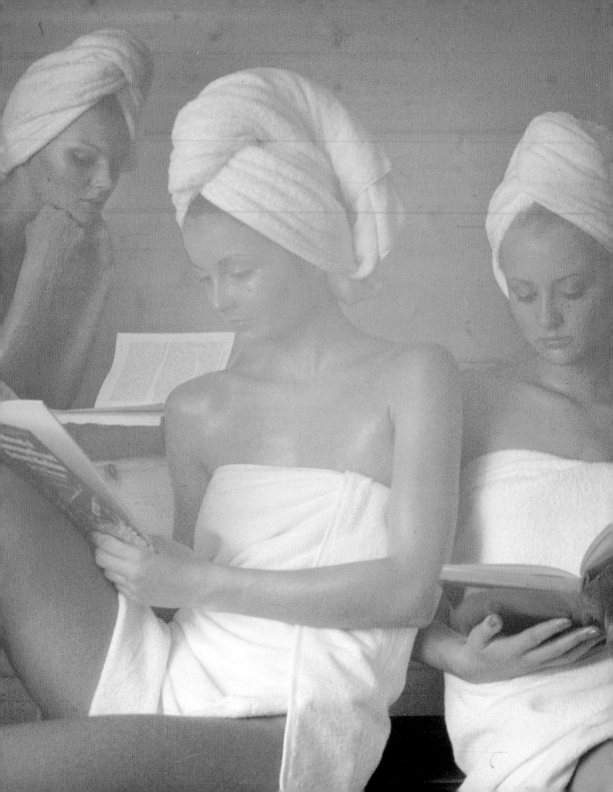

CONTENTS

INTRODUCTION

We all possess the basic ingredients for beauty. And, with the help of experts' superhints and supermodel know-how, beauty is within everyone's grasp. *The Beauty Manual* will show you how.

Let me present the new beauty. She's never had it so good: with cutting-edge cosmetics, accessible high fashion and beauty aids from the fake tan to the Wonderbra, she has all the tools to help her look like she's just stepped off the catwalk. But most importantly she no longer has to conform to the traditional beauty ideal – that hackneyed blueprint of a symmetrical face, big, dewy eyes, a button nose and the body shape of an underfed schoolgirl.

Thanks to the emergence of a new breed of model – who comes in all shapes and sizes – the beauty parameters have broadened. With their crooked noses, buxom bodies, wonky teeth and other so-called 'imperfections', these models have done more for the average woman than Mary Quant's mini did for legs. The message coming loud and clear from the runways is that it's cool to be quirky, hip to be old and beautiful to be big. But this isn't just another fashion moment: there are now as many tastes in beauty as there are types – and they are here to stay!

Read on and rejoice. Modern beauty has little to do with airbrushed perfection and everything to do with accepting your shortcomings and creating a personal beauty style. Just as Barbra Streisand's nose has become her trademark, where would Lauren Hutton be without the cheeky gap between her teeth, or Cameron Diaz without her imperfect, but striking, features? Perhaps the most pertinent example of a celebrity who has not only accepted her so-called 'flaw', but has also turned it into an asset is Cindy Crawford. Take a leaf out of Cindy's book and challenge your beauty identity. You never know, the feature that you hate most about yourself might be the very beauty trait that makes you special.

I believe that everyone has what it takes to be beautiful. Beauty is not an impossible dream, but simply a case of cultivation, both physically and psychologically. We all have the raw materials: even the walking beauty disaster with her half-grown-out, frizz-bomb perm, rampant body hair and brittle, chewed stumps for nails can metamorphose into a head-turning babe to rival any supermodel. Well almost! You see those supermodel paragons of completeness (who are constantly dressed up, made up, pampered and preened) clearly have a head start in the beauty stakes. Yet what really distinguishes models from the rest of us – besides a bevy of image-makers and computer tweaking – is that they have all the tricks of the trade at their fingertips. However, once you have read both the supermodels' and experts' tips revealed in this book, you too will have the advantage of model know-how.

Whether you're in need of a few minor tweaks here and there or a complete image overhaul, every chapter of this book is designed to help you master the art of looking good and maximise your potential. As so many women today live according to a tight schedule, *The Beauty Manual* includes zillions of quick fixes and short cuts to suit low-maintenance beauties. And for the beautyphobe who feels

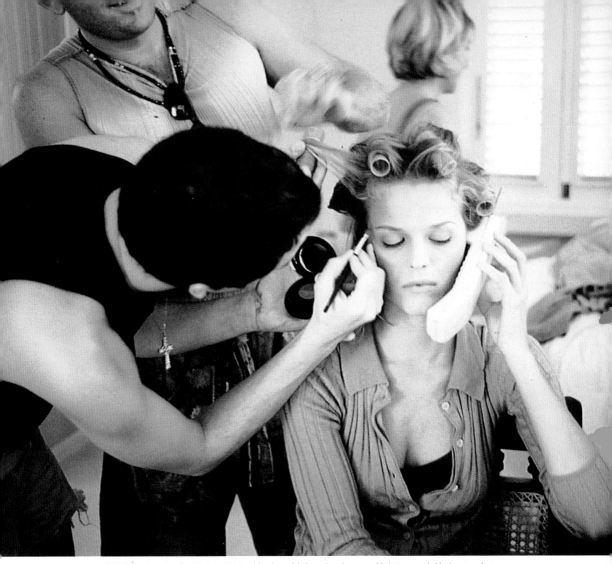

Model know-how: like Eva Herzigova (pictured here), models have the advantage of being surrounded by image-makers.

that visiting the beautician is up there with a trip to the dentist in terms of pleasure, I promise that you won't go short of a few DIY solutions.

The last, yet most important, word in the beauty lexicon is 'confidence'. You may not possess the frame, height or face shape that you desire, but you should learn to love what you have. Regardless of their imperfections, models and celebrities have convinced themselves and others that they are beautiful. You should believe in the philosophy that real beauty power comes from within, that it is a state of mind; for if you think beautiful and act beautiful, you *will* be beautiful. And by the time you turn the final page of *The Beauty Manual*, you should have discovered for yourself that beauty is not in the eye of the beholder, but in the mind, body and spirit of the possessor!

TRICKS OF THE TRADE

Some of the world's leading professionals in the field of beauty – make-up artists, hairstylists, fashion experts, skin specialists, colourists, trichologists, fitness trainers, dieticians and beauty gurus – give their top tips.

For a quick fringe trim, hairstylist to the stars **Oribe's** superhint is: 'Cut only the centre of the bang [fringe] short to guarantee a sexy and perfect bang look.'

'Getting your hair cut regularly every four weeks, even if you only have the ends trimmed, will do more to improve the condition of your hair than anything else,' advises leading international hairdresser **John Frieda**.

World-renowned make-up artist **Mary Greenwell's** top tip is: 'Use lipstick in a multitude of ways – on cheeks and eyes, as well as lips.'

Health and beauty guru **Deepak Chopra's** philosophy is that beauty comes from within, as outlined in this passage from his book *The Path to Love*: 'You are the mirror of divine beauty. Be kind to yourself and others. Come from love every moment you can. Speak of love with others and remember your spiritual purpose. Never give up hope. All people are innocent and beautiful in the light of love.'

'A good treat for your hair is to wash it in Evian water or another good mineral water for two weeks,' says superstylist **Sam Mcknight**. 'You'll be amazed at the difference in the condition of both your scalp and hair.'

Creative director of *Allure* magazine **Polly Mellen** believes that you can learn to dress with style. Her advice is: 'Have a style icon that you admire, and identify what it is about that person that makes he or she stylish.'

Cult perfumer **Jo Malone** has a great party tip: 'Spray a cloud of a couple of your favourite fragrances into the air and walk through it.'

Celebrity colourist **Louis Licari** says: 'No matter what colour you chose to be, I would suggest you stay within a few shades of your natural hair colour: this is usually the most flattering to your skin tone and eye colour. In addition, staying close to your natural hair colour will also make the hair look shiny, vibrant and conditioned.'

Fashion expert **Jo Levin**, who is also the fashion director of *GQ* magazine, gives the following advice for stylish dressing: 'You should be so comfortable with the way you look that you forget what you are wearing. And when buying clothes, find a look that suits your body shape.'

'The whole trick in getting make-up to adhere and last for hours comes down to the layering of creamy (oily or wet) and dry textures,' explains make-up supremo **Bobbi Brown**. 'Concealer, a wet substance, for example, will stay put only if you lock it in place with powder, a dry one.'

'Don't wash your hair,' is the number-one tip from **Orlando Pita**, the stylist behind many of today's catwalk hairstyles, who hasn't shampooed his hair for over a decade and has healthy, shiny tresses to show for it.

'Never underestimate the power of exfoliating,' says **Marcia Kilgore**, owner of the celebrities' favourite urban health spa, Bliss, in New York.

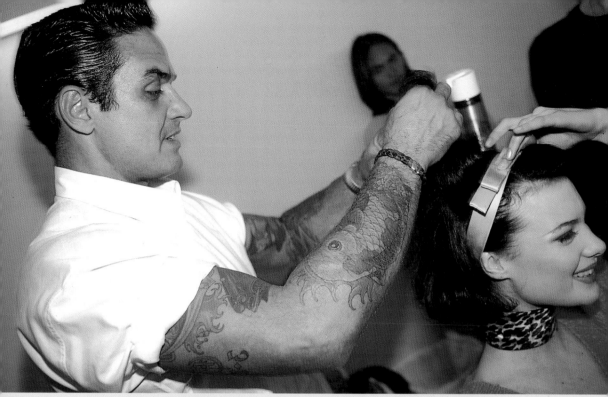

Cartoon cad: stylist to the stars Oribe (pronounced Orbay to those in the know) adds the finishing touches to model Shalom's hair.

If your dark roots are getting you down, the UK's colour doyenne, **Jo Hansford**, has a super tip: 'In-between salon visits, put a little bit of dry-shampoo powder along your parting and dust off any excess. This will defuse the darkness of the roots.'

Trainer to the supermodels **Radu's** advice for a beautiful body is: 'Three to five sessions of organised physical activities per week are imperative. Each weekend must involve some kind of physical activity, such as team sports, nature trips on water, foot or wheels, tennis, squash and outdoor activities such as biking.'

One of beauty guru **Bharti Vyas's** trade secret is: 'Use your hands – they are the best beauty tool.' Bharti is also a great believer in body polishing. 'The secret of healthy skin is polished skin. Exfoliate your body daily and you will have smooth, silky skin and a lean body.'

'For beautiful hair, my number-one tip is simple – wash it daily,' says trichologist to the stars **Philip Kingsley**.

If your hair's fallen flat but you've no time to wash and style it, celebrity hairdresser **Nicky Clarke** has a trick for quick-fix volume and root lift: 'Using heated rollers (either the steam or rubber types, not the ones with plastic spikes that could damage your hair), wind rollers into roots wherever you need the lift. Four or five rollers around the front and crown is probably all you need. Spritz with a fine layer of hairspray, then leave for ten minutes.'

'My top tip is that you shouldn't spend too much time worrying about the way you look. Attempt to be confident and access your features, then enhance them,' says **Millie Kendall**, beauty PR and one of the duo behind Ruby and Millie cosmetics.

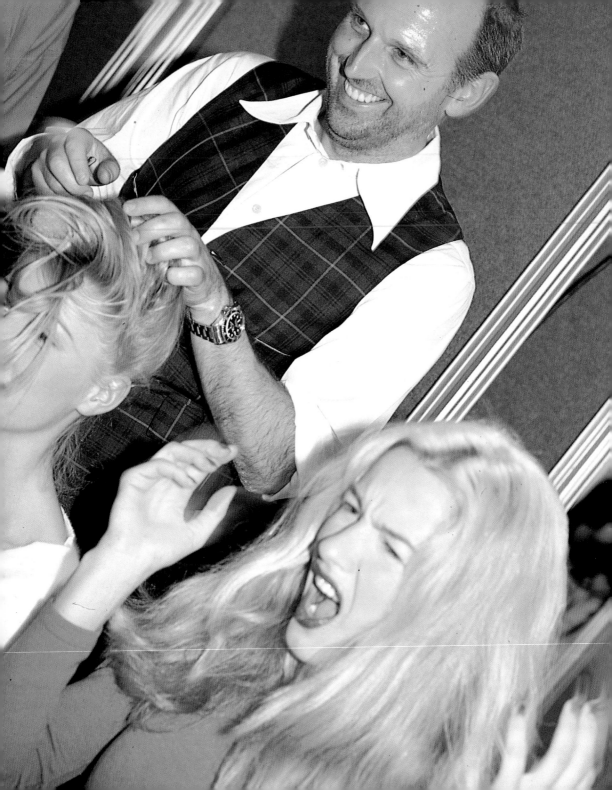

Make-up artist **Ruby Hammer's** top trick of the trade is: 'If you've made any make-up mistakes, e.g. dropped a blob of mascara or splodges of eyeshadow on your face, rather than making a mess by cleansing or smearing, take a Q-Tip [cotton bud], dip it in your foundation and erase the mistake. This also works well for lipstick that is bleeding.'

'Always line your lips after applying lipstick to ensure a perfect shape,' is a tip from world-famous make-up artist **Trish McEvoy**.

For best blow-drying results, award-winning hairdresser **Charles Worthington's** superhints are: 'Rough-dry hair upside down to remove most moisture. Now blow-dry hair in sections – starting from the back underneath, as it's the most time-consuming. Finish blow-drying with a blast of cold air to close the cuticles. When cuticles lie flat, hair reflects the light and looks healthier and shinier.'

Make-up maestro **François Nars'** secret for translating catwalk looks into real life is: 'Catwalk make-up is there to create an "effect". If there is a particular look that inspires you, I recommend that you take just one key element from the look and find a way to work it into your usual look – don't try to reproduce the whole look unless you are going to an occasion where you can carry off the effect.'

Cult skincare specialist **Eve Lom's** top tip is: 'Moderation in drinking, eating and lovemaking – but full speed for cleansing.'

Top make-up artist **Dick Page's** mantra is to ignore the make-up trends and the dos and don'ts: 'Sigourney Weaver has thin lips, yet she wears dark-red lipstick, which is supposedly a no-no. She looks gorgeous and confident. My advice is to wear whatever make-up you feel happy with, not what you're told you should or shouldn't wear.'

'I think actresses are the best women to take inspiration from,' says top make-up artist **Jeanine Lobell**. 'If you can find a look that is versatile, make it work for you. Think of actresses that have similar characteristics to you, and watch carefully how their make-up makes them look in different roles. It might be worth copying a look that you think shows them at their best.'

For healthier eating habits, health columnist and consultant dietician **Lyndel Costain's** advice is: 'Take healthy lifestyle changes a step at a time and be prepared for ups and downs. You'll get there in the end.'

Leading make-up artist **Maggie Hunt** believes that looking great is all down to shaping: 'With make-up, the only way to shape your features is to do so with brushes. This is the key to natural-looking make-up.'

Make-up artist to the stars **Vincent Longo's** great tips for outlining and emphasising eyes are: 'Instead of putting your eyeliner pencil straight onto your eyes, put it onto your hand first, then apply using a flat-headed, quarter-inch, multi-purpose brush. If you want the elongated "cat's-eyes" look, use a pointed lip brush. For longer-lasting effects, apply eyeliner before eyeshadow.'

World-renowned hairstylist **Frédéric Fekkai** believes that in order to get the best possible hairstyle, you have to own a style – a look that will become yours. 'When I see my clients, I always give them tips, not only on haircuts and colour, but on the do's and don'ts about make-up, eyewear and accessories. My philosophy is that the most natural and most simple is the most beautiful. As I always say, don't use make-up to hide your face but use it to show your beauty. Likewise, don't fight the texture of your hair but rather work with it to enhance it.'

Catwalk hairstylist Sam McKnight entertains Karen Mulder (right) and Kirsty Hume (left) to take away some of that backstage boredom.

SUPERMODELS' BEAUTY TIPS

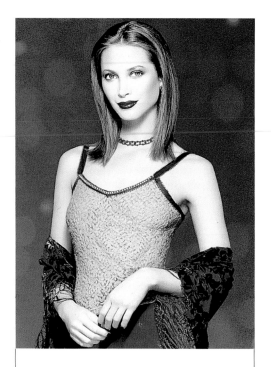

'During the shows, my skin always seems to have a mind of its own, breaking out in everything from acne to eczema, so I need a few little extra somethings,' says **Karen Elson**. 'Aloe vera is probably the best known in skincare, so I mix some of that with vitamin-E oil to give my skin the treat it needs. Origins' Comforting Solution calms my skin and Kiehl's – their products seriously rock and are always handy.'

'I drink lots of water and get a facial once a week, although this is not necessary as once a month should be sufficient,' explains **Caprice**. 'I also cleanse and moisturise every night before I go to bed. Exercise is also very important in order to stay fit, remain healthy and relieve stress.'

Lonneke Engel's tip is: 'Always make sure you clean your face at night before you go to bed'. Her favourite product is Cover Girl's Simply Powder Foundation: 'It gives me a really natural, matte finish.'

Honor Fraser's favourite beauty treatment is spending half an hour or so in a flotation tank: 'It is unbelievably relaxing, which helps maintain a healthy mental state and therefore physical beauty.'

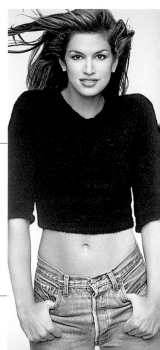

When choosing make-up, **Christy Turlington's** colour preferences are natural browns and neutral shades. She favours a natural look, which she achieves by using such products as Maybelline's Volume Express mascara in Dark Brown and Natural Accents eyeshadows.

Carla Bruni's top tips are to stay out of the sun and not to be obsessive about your looks. For example, she might forget to apply moisturiser one night but she won't fret over it.

Eva Herzigova's skincare routine includes massaging her face every night with her cleansing cream, then removing the cream with a sponge before moisturising her face. On masks, she says: 'If I have any extra time I would rather spend it with friends.'

Cindy Crawford's advice to busy women who want to look good is: 'Try long-wearing products like Revlon's ColorStay hair colours and cosmetics – you'll save time by not having to reapply constantly.'

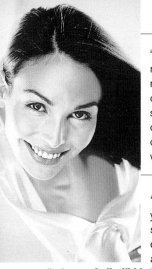

'I try to go to the sauna regularly and put a really nourishing conditioner on my hair before I go in,' says **Inès Sastre**. 'There's one I use by Lancôme called Fluance which works very well.'

'I believe that whatever you put into your body shows on the outside, so I drink lots of water and eat a healthy, well-balanced diet,' says **Jodie Kidd**. 'To escape the suffocating pollution in cities and get fresh air, I go for long country walks. When it comes to what I put on my skin – I'm simply mad about Kiehl's.'

Erin O'Connor's make-up essentials are: 'Always concealer and sometimes a little Aveda mascara.'

'At home I use anything basic or traditional, especially natural-based products by Dr Hauschka, Jurlique, Eve Lom and Jo Malone,' says **Susie Bick** who loves age-old beauty solutions like Chinese herbs and organic products, yet she is fascinated by state-of-the-art salon treatments.

Christie Brinkley's three top tips for looking good are: 'One – smile as much as possible. It has a physiological effect on the body which is uplifting. Two – drink lots of water and eat a varied diet. Three – incorporate different sports into your fitness routine so you don't get tired.'

Veronica Webb's superhints for keeping fit are: 'Whether you do something as simple as stretching before you get out of bed, or dedicate as much as one hour and twenty minutes a day, I think exercise is the most important thing, because no matter how rejected, insecure or bad you feel, it is a way of taking time out for yourself and breaking through those feelings. Exercise says you cherish yourself.'

'For me, it isn't just about losing weight, it's about total well-being – putting time aside for yourself and finding a balance. When you're fit, everything in life is easier to do,' enthuses **Elle Macpherson**.

To keep fit, **Sarah Thomas** swims and cycles. If she were stranded on a desert island, her essential cosmetic would be mascara: 'I like to use a good waterproof mascara in the summer, like Cover Girl's Pro-Aqua Marathon Mascara, which is perfect for hot summer days and nights.'

To relax, **Lucie de la Falaise** soaks in a warm bath sprinkled with sea salt.

Dayle Haddon stays out of the sun: 'I'm religious about it. I wear sunscreen even on my hands, walk on the shady side of the street and I always carry a silk scarf to cover my hair.'

Amber Valetta sticks to a vegetarian diet, drinks plenty of water and takes vitamin supplements. Make-up-wise, she uses her namesake lipstick – Amber – a lip colour created for her by Elizabeth Arden.

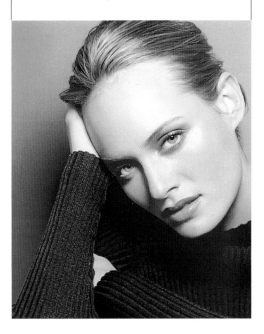

SUPERSTARS' REGIMES

LINDA EVANGELISTA

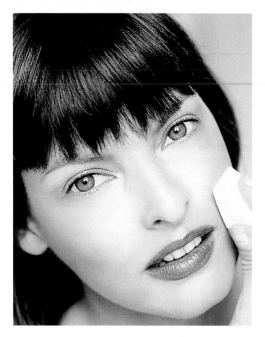

One of the first models to be labelled a 'supermodel', this timeless beauty and talented cook is unquestionably the most beautiful woman I have ever set eyes upon. With her green, cat-like eyes, razor-sharp cheekbones and healthy-looking complexion, it's not surprising that in 1997 she was chosen as the face of cosmetics company Yardley. Here, Linda talks about her make-up 'must-haves' and how she applies them, and gives you some of her make-up tips.

Do you have any tricks of the trade? I don't necessarily wear make-up where it is designed to go. I just love to experiment. I wear lipstick on my cheeks: you have to make sure the skin is well moisturised and the colour's blended carefully with the fingers so the effect is really sheer – it makes for a wonderful, natural, weekend look. (It works better on bare skin than over foundation.) Lip gloss doubles up as a highlighter – try a touch high on the cheekbone and smooth in for a gentle hint of colour. Eye pencils are good for lips: I colour them lightly with Yardley's Eye Definer Pencil in Aubergine and add lip gloss over the top. For a healthy glow, I add a touch of shimmery eyeshadow on my cheekbones.

You have great eyebrows. How do you keep them so well groomed? I tweeze to death. In fact, I have to tweeze every day.

What are your 'must-haves' before you leave the house? My Yardley concealer (my shade is fair), which blends beautifully to disguise any dark circles, and a touch of Brush 'n' Blush. For a really glowing day look, I dust it onto the apples of my cheeks using a fluffy, soft brush. For evening, I stroke it along my cheekbones for a more sophisticated look – starting at the outside and working inwards from the ear. Always, with any blusher, tap the handle of the brush on a hard surface to get rid of any excess before you put it to your face. That's the secret of a natural look.

If you were stranded on a desert island, what would be the beauty essentials that you could not do without? I'd pack an SPF 25 sunscreen, my Yardley Lip Velvet SPF 30 (a really high sun-protection factor) and a brow pencil.

You always look stunning and very natural – do you have any other make-up tips to help the rest of us to look great? To find out whether a lipstick shade suits you, don't try it on the back of your hand; instead, use the tip of one of your fingers, where the colour is closest to lip tone. To give a youthful pout, you can draw slightly outside the natural line, creating two little 'peaks' where the Cupid's bow should be. So long as you always bring the line back perfectly to the edge of the lips it will always look really natural.

JULIETTE BINOCHE

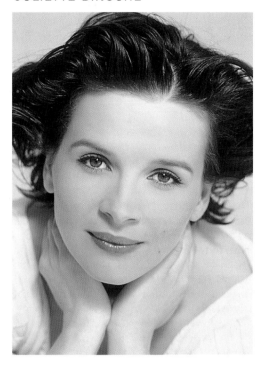

Oscar-winning actress Juliette Binoche received the award for her outstanding role in *The English Patient*. But in October 1995 she was honoured with a different kind of accolade, when she was chosen as the face of Lancôme's new perfume – Poême. Born in Paris in 1964, this great modern actress has that refreshing and very special kind of beauty that goes way beyond the physical – which is exactly why I picked her as one of the world's greatest beauties.

Do you believe that inner beauty is as important as a beautiful exterior? Absolutely. The happier you are the better you look – a beautiful exterior is not enough. Skin is skin, but what makes it special is what people can feel and see. In my work I look for clarity in my thoughts and in my eyes so that people can read what is happening inside, like a book.

Do you have a specific skincare routine? I don't go over the top on beauty products, apart from face creams that stop my skin drying out. I find Lancôme's products really suit my skin.

What is the key to a healthy, radiant skin? I suppose I could say that I owe my career to my skin, but I really don't do much to it. I would say that the key is to breathe correctly, eat lots of fresh fruit and vegetables and drink lots of water.

What are you views on ageing? Ask me again when I'm old! Unlike many other actresses, I'm not scared of getting older. Age shouldn't be an obsession. It's not a question of age but a question of light. If you still have a fire inside you when you're seventy, you'll still be beautiful.

What is your fitness routine? I don't have a special routine. I think people should listen to their bodies and find their own balance.

Do you have any regular complementary therapies? I think massage is the best way to keep happy and healthy. Everyone should learn how to massage – it's an unbeatable way of bonding with someone.

Do you eat healthily? I don't follow any particular diet. However, I eat a healthy mix of foods, including vegetables and salads. If I've overeaten, I drink plenty of water the following day. Talking to a dietician encouraged me to find ways of looking after myself.

Do you have a favourite item of skincare or make-up? I love Lancôme's Hydrative – a velvety daily moisturiser that sinks into my skin, leaving it supple and smooth.

You are the face of Poême; what are your favourite fragrances, and why do you think it is important to wear a fragrance? The single beauty product that I could not live without is perfume. It has a history of seduction and love. You can't change your perfume as easily as you might, say, change a shirt. A smell is much more evocative of a past moment, of a secret. My first perfume was Fidji, a present from my uncle. I've worn fragrances in different phases of my life to correspond to the roles I was playing at the time. In *The Seagull* I wore Poême, and have worn it ever since because it suits me.

What is your beauty philosophy? The best advice I've ever been given is just to be yourself, because if you try to be someone else that's when you start to have problems.

NIKI TAYLOR

Supermodel and supermother of two twin sons, Hunter and Jake, Niki Taylor has that natural, wholesome, all-American look that makes her one of the classic beauties of our day. Her modelling career kicked off to a good start when, at fifteen, she became the youngest-ever model to appear on the cover of *Vogue*. In 1992 Niki achieved another first when she became the youngest model to be placed under an exclusive cosmetics contract with Cover Girl, of whom she is still the face today.

What are your secrets for looking healthy? I exercise, rest, eat healthily and am happy. I get lots of sleep and take care of my skin. I make sure to keep my skin fresh- and natural-looking by cleansing twice a day (especially after photoshoots, when I have a lot of make-up on). Also, especially when travelling, I drink plenty of water.

Do you have any secrets to success regarding your beauty regime? Well, I really don't have any 'secrets' to my beauty regime. I prefer a natural look, so when I'm not working I wear very little make-up.

What are your favourite cosmetics and why? I spend a lot of time outdoors and I never forget my lips! I love Cover Girl's Continuous Colour Self-renewing Lipstick because it is long-lasting yet contains conditioning ingredients that leave my lips looking and feeling soft and smooth whilst retaining moisture, which is so important in the sun. But the best thing of all is that the colour is self-renewing!

What is your best asset and how do you take care of it? I think my best asset is my smile, so I take good care of my teeth, which means proper brushing and regular dental care and cleaning.

What are your beauty essentials? Although I don't wear lots of make-up, especially at the beach, one of my beauty essentials is mascara. Just one quick coat – that's it. Cover Girl's Pro-Aqua Marathon Mascara does the trick. It's waterproof and, as I enjoy scuba-diving and jet-skiing, it's perfect for me – I can say goodbye to 'raccoon eyes'! It stays put until I want to take it off.

How do you keep fit? I keep fit with my trainer by working out regularly, jet-skiing and hydro-sliding.

What do you like or hate about your body? I like my body: it's mine – all 'original' parts.

Any favourite foods? My mum's lasagne, as well as cheeseburgers, milkshakes, pasta, mashed potatoes with gravy, turkey and Coca-Cola.

What do you wear to relax? I love to be comfortable, so I usually wear leggings and a T-shirt or sweatshirt, and my slippers when I'm at home.

What do you like to wear during the day? My daywear is usually jeans or shorts, together with a sweater or shirt and a pair of sandals.

What are your favourite things? The colour blue, Van Halen, my children, my cats, the beach, the sea, getting a tan, my Bronco, dolphins, white tulips, Cover Girl cosmetics, Arizona, Indian jewellery, shoes, animals, sunny days and talking on the phone.

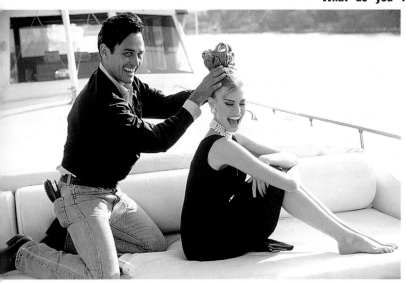

CECILIE THOMSEN

Model-turned-actress Cecilie Thomsen made her acting debut in the Bond movie *Tomorrow Never Lies*. At seventeen this first Danish Bond girl, who hails from a tiny island in Denmark, headed for Paris, where she modelled for such prestigious names as Chanel, Dior and Givenchy, eventually going on to secure a cosmetics contract with Nivea Visage as its new face. Here, this 'drop-dead gorgeous' beauty – as Pierce Brosnan called her – gives readers her top tips.

Do you believe that inner beauty is important? Physical beauty doesn't last very long if the inner beauty is not there. The most beautiful people I know are not supermodels!

What is your best attribute and why? It's difficult to say what you find attractive in yourself as you always tend to pay attention to the negative. If I had to choose something it would be my mouth or my eyes.

Do you have a specific skincare routine and any favourite products, such as treatments or serums? I keep my skin as clean as possible and exfoliate regularly. My favourite beauty product is Elizabeth Arden's Time Capsules, which I use day and night.

Do you ever detox and, if so, how? It's great sometimes when you have a day free to cleanse your system by just eating fruit and drinking freshly-made juices. I find it helps the body rid itself of all its toxins.

What do you wear when you are not on set? On my days off I like to wear no make-up at all to give my skin a rest. If I go out, I use concealer, mascara and lipstick and then I'm ready to go.

How do you relax, and do you have any complementary therapies like shiatsu, acupuncture and so on? When I'm in London, I visit a therapist who clicks my back into place and also does some acupuncture on me. It's a luxury, and helps release any tension in the muscles.

You have a great sense of style; can you describe the type of clothes that you wear? My style is very simple and relaxed. I always choose classic pieces that I can wear for a long time. A

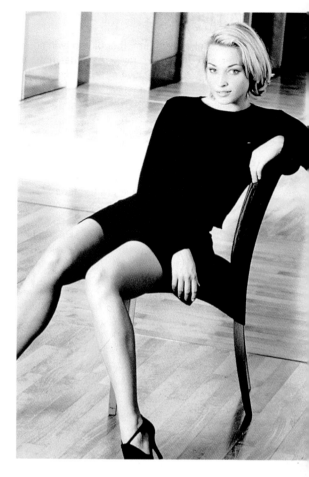

pair of long, narrow pants teamed with a T-shirt is my favourite outfit.

What's your key fitness tip? Try to have fun whilst getting fit. Instead of always doing the same boring routine on the Stairmaster, try kick-boxing, dance, swimming and so on, so that you don't get bored.

What type of foods do you enjoy, and what do you avoid eating? I prefer fresh foods, like fruit salads. I don't like eating fried or processed foods.

What is your philosophy on today's more individual beauty? It is important to see that beauty varies in countless shapes and forms. I wish the fashion magazines would show even more individual beauties.

CELEBRITIES' FAVOURITES

If you want cosmetic kudos, add one or two celebrity favourites
to your make-up bag or beauty cabinet.

Madonna achieves that to-die-for pout with Trucco's Blood Lip Colour.

For naturally glossy lips, **Jodie Kidd** slicks on a smidgen of Clinique's Glosswear and Brush SPF 8 in Air Kiss.

Winona Ryder dabs on Aveda's Love Oil.

Ever wondered what the secret behind **David Ginola's** glossy locks is? He washes them in L'Oréal's Elvive Nutri-Vitamins Shampoo.

Sharon Stone favours Prescriptives' Flight Cream – a fast-working moisture product.

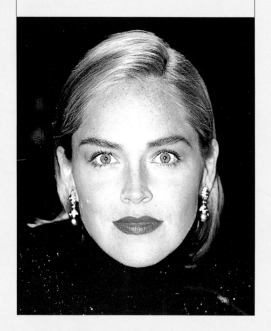

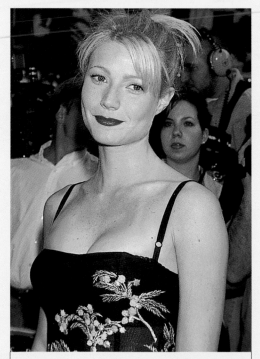

To give her that healthy glow, **Gwyneth Paltrow** uses BeneTint from BeneFits.

When she's on the run, **Susie Bick** wears Max Factor's 3-in-1 Complete Make-up, as it cuts down on application time.

Niki Taylor saves time on lengthy and tricky nail-polish application by painting her nails with Cover Girl's 3-in-1 Nail Sticks.

Uma Thurman uses Cellex-C serum.

To highlight those gorgeous green eyes, **Helena Christensen** uses Shiseido's Liquid Eyeliner.

Naomi Campbell loves to wear MAC's Bardot Satin Lip Colour.

To thicken her lashes, **Meryl Streep** uses Full Potential Mascara in Black/Brown by Clinique.

Paloma Picasso likes Lancôme's Hydrative Moisturiser.

Courtney Cox is a big fan of MAC's Spice Lip Pencil.

Melanie Griffith loves Revlon's Age-defying Foundation.

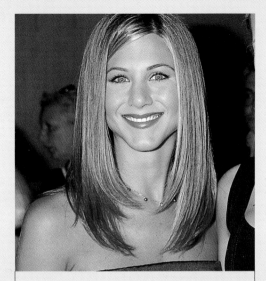

To help create the 'Rachel' hair-do, **Jennifer Aniston** uses L'Oréal's Elvive Mousse.

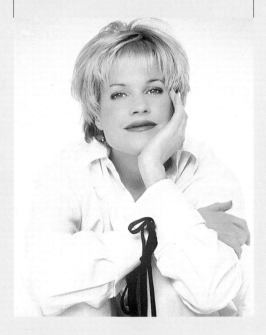

Kate Winslet favours masks from Shiseido.

Courtney Love adores Lightning, by BeneFits, for its shimmery effect.

For a silky-smooth body, **Drew Barrymore** uses Aveda's Smoothing Body Polish.

Like many other supermodels, **Kate Moss** is a big fan of Maybelline's Great Lash Mascara.

Dannii Minogue uses Clarins' Alpine Cleanser.

Revlon's ColorStay Lipstick in Sienna keeps **Cindy Crawford's** lips looking great for hours.

L'Oréal's Rouge Pulp Liquid Lip Gloss is a favourite of **Mila Jovovich**.

To keep her hands silky smooth, **Jade Jagger** buys Dr Hauschka's hand cream.

Elle Macpherson paints her pout with Clinique's Almost Lipstick in Black Honey.

To define her brows, **Tina Turner** uses Lancôme's Crayon Sourcils Eyebrow Pencil.

Michelle Pfeiffer uses Shiseido's Vital Perfection Hydro-Intensive Mask.

Patsy Kensit says that MAC's Lip Glass is the best.

WHAT'S ON A SUPERSTAR'S
BEAUTY SHELF

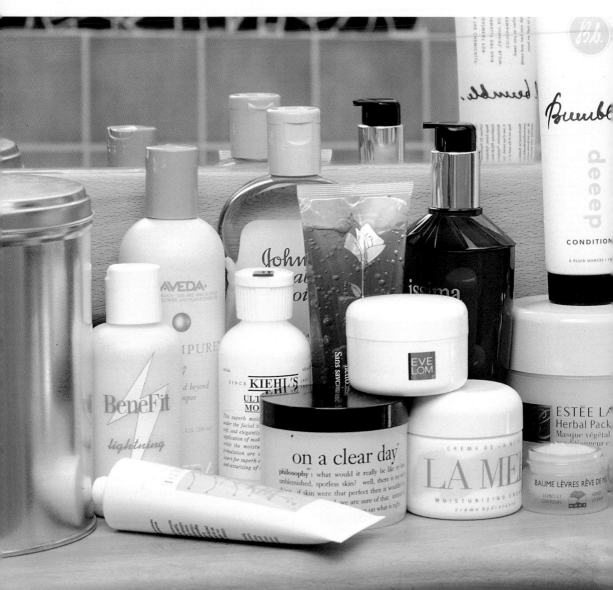

Elle magazine's beauty editor, Rosie Green, lets us into one of her best-kept secrets: what supermodels and celebrities keep on their bathroom beauty shelves.

Aveda's Shampure • Bumble and Bumble's Deep Conditioner • Origins' Salt Body Scrub • Nuxe's Honey Lip Balm • Johnson's Baby Oil • Lancôme's Gentle Cleansing Foaming Gel • Remède's Sweep • Crème De La Mer • Philosophy's On a Clear Day • Tweezerman's tweezers • Alka-Selzer • Razors • Winnie the Pooh plasters • Guerlain's Issima Bodysérum • Estée Lauder's Herbal Pack Conditioner • Eve Lom's Day Cream • Cotton buds • Tony and Tina's Nail-varnish Remover • Eau D'Hadrien, by Annick Goutal • Clarins' Eau Dynamisante • Kiehl's Ultra Facial Moisturiser • BeneFits' Lightning • Clinique's Turnaround Cream

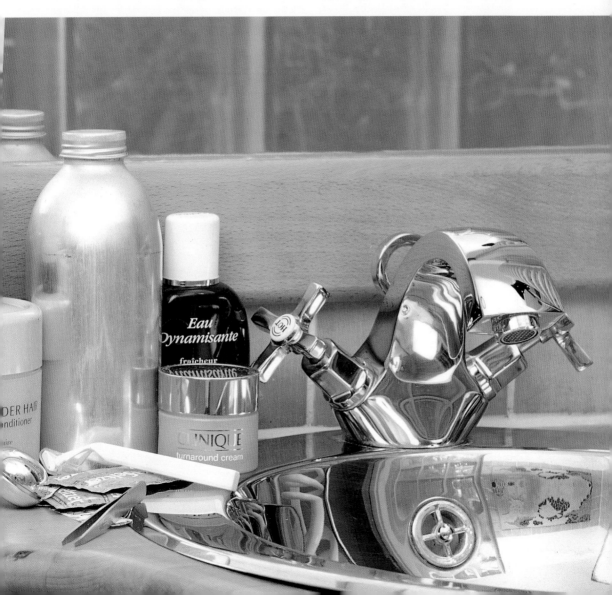

WHAT IS BEAUTY?

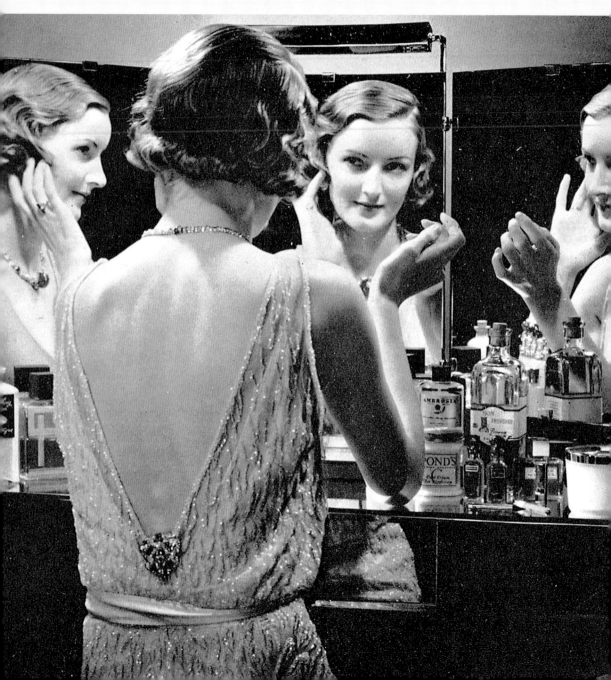

Beauty is a hot commodity, but what is this intangible quality?

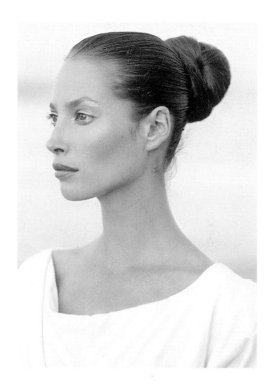

We all want to be beautiful. We may nibble at our unlacquered nails, neglect our skin and nonchalantly say that we don't give a damn, but deep down we desire to look like the ravishing supermodels that stare out at us from every news-stand, TV screen and advertising hoarding.

The quest for beauty doesn't plague Western society alone: it's a global phenomenon and a primal one, too. In the African bush, for example, tribeswomen use face paint to beautify themselves, and while Japanese geishas whiten their faces with powder, their Indian sisters are busily decorating their bodies with henna.

For centuries, us mortals have been beautifying ourselves and, what's more, have suffered to be beautiful. In the 1500s, for instance, British men and women risked lead poisoning by painting their faces with ceruse – a lethal mixture of white lead and vinegar. During the Cold War, Soviet women would save their ration cards to buy the ubiquitous blue eyeshadow. And, apparently impervious to the discomfort, some Papua New Guinea tribeswomen sting their breasts with nettles so that they swell up; Ethiopian Surma tribeswomen have their lower lips stretched and a six-inch plate inserted; and many women from Sudanese, Nigerian and other African tribes scar their skins for decorative purposes.

Why is appearance so important to us, and why is such a high value placed upon it? Perhaps it's because we believe that good looks win the choicest prizes: everything from

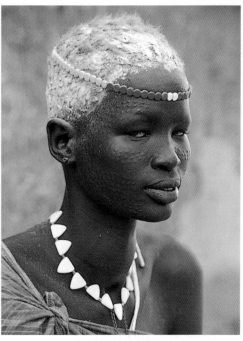

Left: 1930s beauty surrounded by the most popular elixirs of the era – cold cream and perfume.
Above: Classic Western beauty. Supermodel Christy Turlington has been hailed the most beautiful woman of our time and was awarded the title 'Face of the 20th Century' by New York's Metropolitan Museum of Art.
Right: Nuet tribeswoman. Elaborate scars and face paint are the chief beautifiers for tribeswomen.

popularity at school to Hollywood contracts. We are now living in aesthetically literate times, where appearance does matter, and to go unnoticed is akin to being invisible.

The notion of beauty is learned very early on: according to Nancy Friday, in her book *The Power of Beauty* (Hutchinson, 1996), pretty babies get picked up first. It's a natural instinct to be drawn to things that please the eye, which is why children become aware of prettiness at such an early age, associating ugliness with 'baddies' and beauty with the good and kind. (Think of Disney heroines, aren't they invariably beautiful?)

A thing of beauty is a joy for ever:
Its loveliness increases; it will never
Pass into nothingness . . .

John Keats (1795–1821),
Endymion (1818).

Look up the word 'beauty' in any dictionary and you'll find a list of definitions as long as your arm. Yet how is it quantified? Radu, fitness trainer to the stars, defines the general acceptance of a beautiful body as: one, physical appearance – proportions, dimensions and definition; colour (pigmentation) of the skin, hair and eyes; form of the nose and lips; two, abilities – how you move; agility; performance and grace; and three, forces – energy; sexual attractiveness; magnetism; brain energy; mental attitude; intelligence; alertness; culture; and manners.

Some scientists claim that beauty is quantifiable purely by means of facial symmetry: if the space between your eyes, the length of your nose and width of your mouth measure up to their specifications, you pass the beauty test. There is even an Internet website that uses a similar method to evaluate from a snapshot whether you are ugly, average, attractive or beautiful. But this type of scientific formula is questionable, for if symmetry did equal beauty, some of today's models, with their widely-spaced eyes or crooked noses, wouldn't even have made it through their model-agencies' doors, let alone have been considered beautiful.

Furthermore, mathematics cannot explain why what is considered ravishingly beautiful in some cultures is often deemed ugly in others. Eskimos and African tribesmen, for example, typically prefer a large-hipped woman with facial scars and droopy breasts to a stick-thin supermodel. So not only is beauty subjective, but it is also subject to cultural ideals. However, with the world fast becoming a global village and models being recruited from every corner of the world, the Western perception of beauty is changing. When supermodel Alek Wek (see picture on page 149), from the Sudanese Dinka tribe, became the face of Issey Miyake, Joop, Moshino and Clinique, it was clear that the Western world had at last begun to accept even the strongest racial look as beautiful.

Beauty and youth

For years, egged on by the media, Western society worshipped youth. Today, however, the media has readjusted its notion of beauty to accept that the mature woman can be gorgeous, rather than simply dismissing her when she reached her 'sell-by' date. The current acceptance of older models isn't merely a temporary respite from the relentlessly young model army. Advertisers who once clung to the under-twenties to promote their products now use women of forty and over. We must salute the likes of Lauren Hutton, Isabella Rossellini, Catherine Deneuve and Carmen Dell'Orefice who secured top advertising campaigns in their forties, fifties and sixties, and who have shown the world that beauty doesn't fade – it matures.

Beauty and size

The size issue has plagued us like no other. Richard Klien, author of *Eat Fat* (Picador, 1996), has predicted that as we enter the post-modern age we will begin to love fat. This hasn't happened – yet. Nonetheless, not since Rubenesque-style curves were the height of fashion has our culture been so against dieting: you can't open a newspaper without reading column inches about anorexia or articles dedicated to ridiculing the latest so-called 'miracle' diet. Encouragingly, larger actresses and models are stepping into the limelight. Far from being out of shape, these women are proud of their bodies and are proof that big is beautiful.

Beauty and brains

'Bimbo': this was the word coined for women who were attractive but not clever. The bimbo was said to be too busy filing her nails and bleaching her hair to read a broadsheet newspaper or have an intellectual conversation. This stigma may have arisen from the collective envy of beautiful people on the part of those who were lacking in the looks department. But the fact that Christy Turlington read philosophy at Columbia University, Sharon Stone has an exceptionally high IQ, Inès Sastre speaks four languages and Geena Davis is a member of Mensa, shows that beauty can go hand in hand with brains. So rather than swap your stilettos for more sensible shoes, be confident that you can be attractive and still have a discussion on literature or the state of the economy for that matter.

Modern beauty

During the Renaissance, such paintings as *Primavera* (c. 1477) by Botticelli and *The Judgment of Paris* (c. 1600) by Rubens, which depicted voluptuous women, set the style. From the twentieth century onwards, it was the media 'Über-powers' (magazine fashion editors and photographers) who dictated what was beautiful.

Until recently, one particular look would dominate an era: in the 1950s it was the Bardot-style, hour-glass figure, while in the 1960s the look was personified by the cigarette-thin, doe-eyed Twiggy, later followed by the high-gloss supermodels of the early 1990s. Then towards the late nineties this trend changed and the widest variety of beauties came traipsing down the catwalk, including the ginger-bobbed Karen Elson who, with her quirky face, small eyes and sparse eyebrows, was living confirmation that the modern beauty is idiosyncratic and not a mathematical equation. Pleased to be free of earlier boundaries, make-up maestro François Nars proclaims that there is not just one type of beauty today. This philosophy is echoed by Bobbi Brown, leading make-up artist and author: 'There is no one "perfect" beauty standard but countless expressions of personalised beauty.'

The essence of modern beauty is all about having the right outlook. Instead of getting hung up over her imperfections, today's beauty resolves to turn her flaws into assets. Having accepted her fundamental body shape, height, age, racial origin and facial features, she is comfortable with herself. What's more, she realises the importance of striking a healthy balance: working hard at making the very best of herself, without being totally obsessive, she makes sure that she doesn't lose either her lust for life or inner sparkle – both crucial facets of modern beauty.

With her quirky looks, model Karen Elson proves that modern beauty is idiosyncratic and not a mathematical equation.

CHECKLIST FOR BEAUTY

If dogs bark at you and babies cry when you pass them in the street, there's
no need to stick a paper bag over your head. Everyone has the potential to look good
locked within them. Here is a handy checklist to help you kick start the beautifying process.

• **Think of your image as a whole:** Rather than concentrating on one element, regard each aspect of your appearance as a piece of a jigsaw that you need to slot together in order to get the whole picture. Your hair and make-up are linked to your clothes, accessories and shoes, for example, and are all part of the total image composition.

• **Visualise the new you:** Shut your eyes and imagine yourself looking stunning in a little black party number or a tiny bikini, or envisage the looks on your colleagues' faces when they see a sexier, slimmer you. Keep positive images such as these in your mind while you exercise, eat healthily and exfoliate in working towards your goal.

• **Assess your motivation for change:** Ideally, you should want to look great for yourself. But if that reason does little to motivate you, you may find that another motive – whether it be to entice your ideal partner or clinch that dream job – helps push you towards striving to become more beautiful.

• **Work out your weaknesses:** Stand in front of a full-length mirror, with a second mirror angled so that you can see your front, back and sides. Decide what aspect of your appearance needs improving and think about ways in which you can improve it. If it's your bottom that's a minus point, for instance, start exercising and invest in clothes that slim down your derrière.

• **Don't fret over minor flaws:** If you spend all your time worrying about a minor imperfection like a spot, stretchmark or wrinkle you will end up visualising the problem as being far worse than it actually is.

• **Draw up a plan of ways to reinvent yourself:** Write down all the things that you need to do in order to transform yourself: for instance, clear out your wardrobe, get you teeth fixed, make an appointment to have your hair coloured or visit a beauty counter to update your make-up. And, don't forget to take the whens, wheres and hows into consideration.

• **Don't be defeatist:** When you embark on a new exercise routine or skincare regime be patient, or else you will find yourself giving up before you have had the chance to reap any benefits. Once you notice that your skin is glowing and your body is toning up, you will need no other motivation to keep going.

• **Playtime:** Set aside an evening to play around with your make-up, hair and clothes. Work on improving your image and aim to create a couple of new looks.

• **Feel good about yourself:** Positive thinking towards the way you look will have a dramatic effect on your morale and self-confidence.

• **Look well groomed:** Having beauty intelligence means paying attention to the nitty gritty details. For instance: keep your nails neat, remove unwanted facial or body hair, and check for such clothing discrepancies as missing buttons and hanging hemlines.

• **Make five new beauty resolutions:** Resolve that over a certain period (a week, month or six months from now, perhaps), you will introduce into your life five new – realistically achievable – steps towards improving your looks. For example: resolve to floss your teeth every night, introduce healthier foods into your diet, do facial exercises, start skin-brushing.

NEW AGE HOLISTIC BEAUTY

'Mind, body and spirit' and 'holistic' are the current beauty catch phrases which, when translated from beauty speak into everyday language, mean beautifying and caring for ourselves from the inside out: allowing the mind, body and spirit to work in unison.

Beauty guru and author of *Beauty Wisdom* (Thorsons, 1998), Bharti Vyas – whose disciples include Belinda Carlisle, Sophie Dahl and Ralph Fiennes – is just one of the many beauty professionals who believe in the concept of the integrated whole. 'The key to beauty is inner health achieved through nutrition, massage to cleanse the lymphatic system, good posture, correct breathing and exercise to keep your face and body in shape,' says the woman who mixes traditional therapies with state-of-the-art technology.

The approach of age-old Eastern beauty therapies has always been a holistic one, so it comes as no surprise that traditional therapies have found a place within the modern beauty philosophy. Eastern remedies, principles and treatments, such as Ayurveda – an ancient healing system from India – are fast becoming as popular in the Western world as the more conventional beauty treatments. Being beaten with birch twigs one minute and having a microcurrent facial the next may sound like a bizarre combination, but they complement each other and result in beauty harmony.

Looking and feeling great means addressing mental and emotional well-being as well as the physical. With slogans like 'clear mind, clear skin' inscribed on their bottles, even cosmetics companies are marketing the fact that the mind affects the body and the way we look. Bharti stresses that if you are unhappy at work or in your love life, your external appearance will suffer. In pursuit of her aim to help women understand that beauty is about more than just drenching your skin in face cream, Bharti has designed a 'beauty clock' which charts how beauty is linked to, or affected by, such factors as emotions, diet, habits, lifestyle and stress. Having done the 'beauty-clock test', take the holistic approach towards beauty and you will soon find your own beauty equilibrium.

BHARTI'S BEAUTY CLOCK

EMOTIONS
- Am I happy and satisfied in work?
- Am I happy and satisfied in my lovelife?
- Do I express my emotions in a healthy authentic way?

DIET
- Do I eat plenty of fresh fruit and vegetables?
- Do I keep wheat and dairy to a well-managed minimum?
- Do I check my diet and change it when I need to?

MEDICATION
- Do I keep an eye on my health and prevent rather than need to cure?
- Do I usually use natural remedies?
- Do I cleanse my system after using medications?

AGE
- Am I aware of what to expect at my age in terms of skin conditions and health factors?
- Do I know how to make the best of myself?
- Do I express my emotions in a healthy authentic way?

LIFESTYLE
- Do I do regular exercise?
- Do I balance work, rest and play well?
- Do I check my lifestyle and change it when I need to?

STRESS
- Do I work sensible hours?
- Do I have a de-stressing routine?
- Do I have help and support to keep stress well managed?

HABITS
- Do I have a daily skin care routine?
- Do I do enough for my health and wellbeing?
- Do I notice bad habits and manage them out?

Answer *'Yes'*, *'No'* or *'To some extent'* to each question. Every *'Yes'* counts for **2 points** *'To some extent'* is **1 point**

Scores: 0–14 Call the helpline (00 44 (0)171 486 7910). **15–28** Not bad – room for improvement. **29–42** Congratulations – keep it up!

INNER BEAUTY

Beauty goes infinitely deeper than face value, so if you want to improve your looks focus on your inner glow.

Charm, vibrancy and magnetism: these qualities are sparked by something far more compelling than the colour of your hair or your face shape. Cosmetics, clothes, exercise and diet all play their part in creating good looks, but it is inner beauty that takes the major role in the big beauty picture. This priceless beauty ingredient is invincible, transcending time and all the other factors that affect our physical appearance. If an internal fire glows within, it manifests itself outwardly as glistening eyes and a dazzling smile.

If you find the concept of inner beauty hard to grasp, try to imagine how someone who lacks it might be: an expressionless person who does not sparkle, whose smile is forced and who has little or no personal aura or charisma. I have met many women and men who might be considered physically unattractive if it wasn't for their inner beauty. One such person that springs to mind is an overweight man whose charm and lust for life give him more presence than the most drop-dead-gorgeous Adonis. Another is a relatively ordinary-looking woman, whose sparkling eyes and radiant, smiling face impart her with natural beauty.

But before you chuck out your make-up and mutter a prayer of thanks for this thing called 'inner beauty', don't think that relying on it means that you can neglect your exterior. Treat it like that of a car – a material object that you want to keep polished, regularly serviced and take pride in. Remember, however, that it is the engine and the person driving the car that really matter, so develop your inner glow, too, and you will embody a very special package indeed.

Happiness equals beauty

Happiness has a powerful effect on both your inner and outer beauty. Cristina Carlino, founder of the New Age cosmetics company Philosophy, whose products treat both the psyche and the skin, believes that if a woman is unhappy she will never feel beautiful: 'I believe that beauty comes from within', says Cristina. 'It is a woman's warmth and personality shining out that makes her beautiful, not the colour of her eyes. Unhappiness will ultimately show in her face and expressions.'

A truly beautiful person is someone with a warm heart, who is kind, generous and caring, as these are the essential nutrients for the soul. On the flip side, bitterness, envy, jealousy, criticism, tension and other negative feelings and emotions reveal themselves in the face and can mar both inner and outer beauty. Strive to be as happy as possible and do things that induce positive moods such as laughing, listening to music, watching a good film and spending time with friends.

Happiness smoothes out the rough edges in your mind; notice how when you are happy your frown lines vanish and a softer expression appears on your face. Because, at the end of the day, happy thoughts are more effective than the most expensive beauty treatment.

Beauty is an attitude

I can munch salad like a rabbit, say 'no' to cigarettes and meditate nearly as well as any Buddhist, but the one element of beauty that I, and many others, find difficult to master is the mind. You feel young, but your mind keeps telling you that you're old; you've been told that you're attractive, yet your mind won't accept it. Such destructive thoughts result in self-criticism, which can spiral into low self-esteem. A healthy mind is intrinsically linked to inner beauty and is also vital for a positive self-image and self-confidence. So work hard at thinking positively and at obliterating any negative thoughts; you'll soon find that your mind and body will become harmonised.

Show enthusiasm and interest in life

One infallible way of increasing your inner glow is to show interest in both others and everything going on around you – world events, your job, your city and your friends. And whether it's a mundane chore or something more riveting, be enthusiastic about everything that you do and your facial expressions will always be animated. Vibrancy, warmth and beauty emanate from someone who has enthusiasm and is interested in life.

Smile!

People fall in love with a smile – it makes you look twice as pretty and knocks years off your age. Smiling is incredibly infectious and has a habit of winning people over. A warm smile and radiant expression can invest even the plainest person with beauty. But remember there is a big difference between a natural smile that stems from your heart, and a superficial grin that is forced or insincere.

Let your eyes sparkle

Eyes light up a face. Often referred to in literature as the windows of your soul, they speak volumes about your inner thoughts, feelings and emotions. Notice how people's eyes sparkle when they are enthusiastic and become dull when they are sad. No amount of eyeliner, eyeshadow or mascara can bring a natural twinkle to the eyes in quite the same way that inner beauty can. Sparkling eyes make your whole expression come alive, so look people in the eye, talk with your eyes and, most importantly, smile with your eyes.

Loosen up your body language

Inner beauty – or the lack of it – not only shows in your facial expressions, but is also apparent in your body movements, gesticulations and poise. If you hold your body stiffly, hunch over, tense your hands and fidget, you will look awkward and will prohibit your inner beauty from shinning through. Aim to keep your body relaxed. Check your posture and watch that your shoulders are not hunched up: to release tension, shrug shoulders and shake hands and legs.

Don't become obsessive

Obsessions with exercising and calorie-counting, as well as overly-rigid beauty routines, can destroy your inner glow. Don't become too preoccupied with your appearance or you will probably end up boring both yourself and those around you. Break your routine once in a while: guzzle a bar of your favourite chocolate at the weekend; skip exercise while on holiday; and intentionally forget to apply your superserum anti-ageing cream.

Cultivate your personality

Personality plays a major role in the inner-beauty picture. It is often said that some very beautiful people rely solely on their looks to get them friends, jobs, partners and so on. But looks are ephemeral and the vacuous beauty will eventually become unstuck.

By way of an example, I remember having lunch with a young, up-and-coming model who had just won an international contest and was consequently in great demand with some of the world's most prestigious magazines and photographers. I asked her what her parents thought of her new-found modelling career and in her response she implied that she couldn't be bothered to answer such a boring question. In fact, I later learned that this precocious babe thought that she was *so* outstanding that she was above speaking to anyone – including other models, her booker and even her clients. Having previously admired her beauty, I was then amazed at how quickly her flawless skin, razor-sharp cheekbones, big, blue eyes and long legs seemed to lose their allure.

CONFIDENCE

Confidence is your number-one beauty asset: it's sexy, sassy and smart.
Learn to shine with confidence and not only will everyone think that you're gorgeous,
but I guarantee that you'll be one of life's winners.

Confidence – the chief beautifier – is possibly the most elusive asset of all: you won't find it on sale at the cosmetics counter, designer boutique or even a swanky hair salon. Admittedly, a fabulous new frock or a revamped hair-do might act as a temporary booster, but image changes do not give you true confidence, the type that does not require the sanction of others and is strong enough to overcome any number of knocks.

Our confidence levels often fluctuate, rather like a barometer, moving to sunny when we know that we look good or receive a compliment, and getting stuck in a depression when we are suffering from a bout of insecurity. Confidence is a mind-body connection: it's about self-belief and being comfortable with your looks regardless of your shortcomings. Many of us are guilty of putting ourselves down and getting depressed about our flaws, no matter how attractive we are. Even a bad-hair day can shatter our confidence, quite apart from agonising over our large thighs or big nose, say, to which we apportion the blame for practically everything that is wrong in our lives. But remember: beauty is merely about giving an impression, so give the impression that you are content and confident with your looks and not only will the rest of the world think you are gorgeous but, most importantly, you'll start believing it, too.

We've all turned green with raw envy when a lissom Elle Macpherson lookalike strolls across our path with an air of elegant self-assurance. You may feel like poking her in the eye with your lip brush, but bear in mind that true confidence has little to do with 'in-your-face' good looks. Confidence alone is attractive. (If you've ever admired someone's appearance yet had difficulty pinpointing a tangible beauty attribute, you'll understand what I mean.)

One girl illustrated to me what true confidence is all about. Word spread that a friend had met a beautiful woman. On meeting Georgina, my model-agent-trained eye searched for some feature or aspect of her appearance that I could classify as beautiful. Admittedly she entered the room like a seasoned celebrity and had pretty, bob-length red hair, but her features were relatively ordinary, her lips were small and her chin protruded. I was silently calling my friends blind when it hit me: this girl had something magnetic – she exuded an aura of natural self-confidence. I was intrigued with finding out where Georgina's enduring confidence stemmed from. As I spent more time in her company, it became apparent that she had been treated like a goddess from day one. Having quickly learned to love herself from an early age, she had high self-esteem and self-value – a precious gift that she will undoubtedly carry with her for the rest of her life.

Neuro Linguistic Programming (NLP) teacher Jean Pain, who is also an author of self-help books, believes that our upbringing plays a vital role in confidence-building. 'We are all born confident,' says Jean. 'I have yet to find a baby

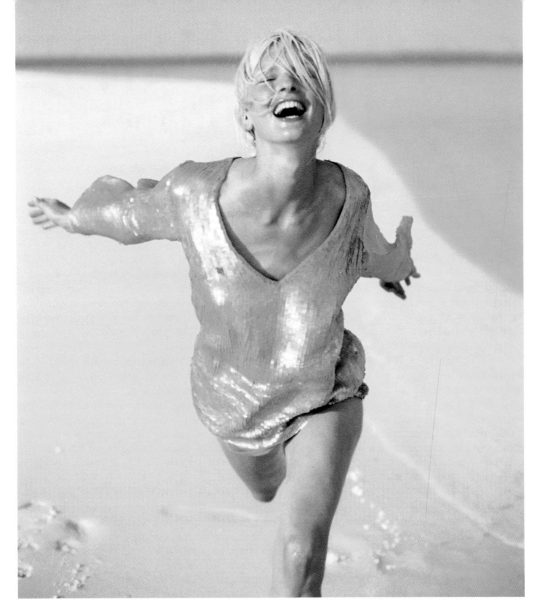

lacking confidence. It's outside influences that cause our confidence to get shaken'. Jean has counselled many clients who hated the way they looked and lacked confidence, even though they were physically gorgeous. 'A distorted self-image is not dissimilar to anorexia,' Jean points out. 'When these people look in the mirror they don't see a correct image of themselves. It's as if their beauty is invisible. Many spend so much time comparing themselves with someone else, they lose their own sense of identity.'

At the end of the day, if you don't like yourself no amount of image-tweaking will give you confidence. Therefore, the first lesson in becoming more self-confident is to learn to love yourself.

A DOZEN WAYS IN WHICH TO BOOST YOUR CONFIDENCE

If you were at the back of the queue when confidence was handed out, here are a few pointers that will help you become a more confident person.

1 Tell yourself that you are unique

There is no one else on earth who is quite like you, so don't compare yourself with others. Wishing that you looked different, or like a friend or actress you admire, will not change anything – you will just end up going through life being miserable. Besides, the modern beauty does not slavishly copy: she is proud to be herself and has her own sense of identity.

2 Act as if you are confident

If you do so, not only will others believe that you are confident, but you'll start to become more self-assured, too. For a young actor, model, athlete, musician or politician who has just been thrust into the limelight, it is imperative that they project an aura of confidence, even if they are a shrinking violet underneath. If you observed the progress of such a person, you'd notice how, after a few months in the business, the façade is replaced with enduring confidence.

3 Walk with confidence

Good posture and carriage will instantly label you confident and gives others the impression that you are proud of yourself (see page 166). Try this exercise when you next enter a room full of people: hold your head higher and walk taller – now notice how heads turn!

4 Transform your confidence by revamping your image

Buying as little as just one item of clothing, which will enable you to create a whole new outfit, can work wonders, as can sporting a great new hairstyle (provided you don't make a rash decision to have it all cut off or bleached blonde: a bad hair mistake could plummet your confidence levels to even greater depths). As for your body: if you need to shed a few pounds, start exercising and following a healthy-eating plan – the motivation alone will increase your confidence.

5 Build up a positive self-image

Firstly, don't allow another's comment to undermine your self-image. Many people base their self-image on a remark that someone made two months or even two decades ago. If this is the case and it is still bothering you, try telling it to a friend or counsellor – you'll soon release how petty it sounds. And remember, people who criticise others tend to be unhappy with themselves. Secondly, be aware that the reflection you see in the mirror has a dramatic influence on your self-image. If you spend every day in sloppy old leggings and a baggy jumper, you will get so used to seeing yourself as a frump that this vision will become your self-image. So dress well – for yourself as well as others.

6 Hype yourself up

Start by identifying your physical plus points and then bombard yourself with compliments. Say to yourself 'I am gorgeous and sexy; I do have beautiful eyes, long legs, white teeth and a cracking smile.' As well as hyping up your external assets, praise your work and value your personality highly, and you will soon find that any self-doubt is replaced by self-belief and greater self-confidence.

7 Boost your self-esteem with a list

Grab several sheets of paper and prepare to write the following lists:

- all your physical plusses i.e. eyes, lips, skin, hair, legs;
- everything that you have achieved in your life (this could include things like buying a house or car, passing exams, learning a language, having a child);
- all the things that you are good at, like sports, dancing, public-speaking, organising events and so on;
- all your personality traits i.e. kindness, generosity, thoughtfulness, ability to make others laugh.

Having compiled your lists, constantly remind yourself of your assets, achievements and skills. If you have any tangible proof of your talents, such as paintings, photographs or certificates, surround yourself with them.

8 Overcome your self-consciousness

Whether you are painfully shy or occasionally blush in public, you are probably self-conscious and therefore lack confidence. Shyness can be overcome with therapy or by reading self-help books, but you can put an instant end to embarrassing blushing by applying a green-tinted primer or skin tint that will tone down any high colour. In order to come across as being more confident and less self-conscious, use eye contact: while downcast eyes scream shyness, looking people directly in the eye imparts confidence.

9 Don't draw attention to your negative points

Keep any negative thoughts to yourself. It's unlikely that your partner or friends will even have noticed your so-called 'flaws', but if you start complaining about how big your bottom is or how much cellulite you have, you'll end up drawing attention to them. And, rather than getting hung up over your body blips, focus on your good points: for example, what silky skin or pert breasts you've got.

10 Find a new focus

Take up a new interest, such as a sport, enrol in an evening class, learn a language or spend more time doing something that you are good at. If you feel confident in this activity you will be proud of your achievements and your overall self-esteem will grow. Focusing on something new will also prevent you from allowing your identity to be governed by your looks.

11 Compose yourself

Get your appearance, home, office and mind in order. This not only gives the impression to others that you are a 'together' type of person, but also gives you the feeling of being in control of different aspects of your life and will therefore empower you with confidence.

12 Try courses or therapies

If your self-confidence is at an all-time low, consider an assertiveness course. Another successful confidence-bolster is a form of self-development (both group and one-to-one) known as Neuro Linguistic Programming, which teaches you how to develop a more positive self-image and hone your social skills. Alternatively, you could try Gestalt, a self-development method of psychotherapy devised by Freudian psychoanalyst Fritz Perls. Practised since the 1950s, it is ideal for people who lack self-esteem or find it difficult to express themselves. If your lack of confidence is deep-rooted, psychotherapy may help.

THE MIRACLE MAKE-OVER

Supermodels reinvent themselves every season, but we ordinary mortals could benefit from the occasional revamp, too. From a sexier walk to a body, hair, make-up and fashion overhaul, this transformation plan is designed to change even the plainest Jane into a sublime beauty – fast.

FACE MAKE OVER

Brighten your eyes

Refresh your eyes by covering them with a chilled eye mask or cucumber slices. • Brighten dull eyes with whitening eye drops. • To highlight and lift your eyes, draw a fine line above the lashes of your upper eyelid (taking it out slightly at corners), and sweep pale eyeshadow such as ivory across your brow bone. • Top make-up artist Ruby Hammer, who has her own range, gives the following tips for stunning, fresh-looking eyes: 'Apply concealer mixed with a tiny dollop of eye cream to under-eye area. To add definition, regardless of the colours you choose, always go for a light, neutral beige/ivory hue on the brow bone, a medium tone on the eyelids and a darker, defining shade close to your lashes'.

Luscious lashes

Thick, dark, curly eyelashes emphasise the eyes more than any amount of eye make-up and add glamour even to the most bare-faced. • Curl your eyelashes with eyelash curlers. For extra hold, try the heated version. • For a longer-lasting curl, have your eyelashes permed at a beauty salon: this not only curls lashes but also lifts them from the roots and really opens up the eyes. • Dye your lashes with a home eyelash-dye kit or visit a salon. • Thicken lashes by dusting them with powder before applying mascara. • Create the impression of fuller eyelashes by dotting a tiny amount of eyeliner pen along your lash line. • To prevent your lashes breaking, condition with Vaseline Petroleum Jelly or Mavala's Double Lash.

Frame your face

Eyebrows deserve as much attention as eyes, so sculpted brows are a must. Shaping and tinting eyebrows can make an enormous difference to your eyes, features and facial shape. • Forget about having to match your brow colour to your hair colour: a couple of shades darker or lighter could really emphasise your eyes. • If you suffer from sparse brows, either define them with an eyeshadow, brow pencil or, alternatively, tint them with an eyebrow-dye kit. • Tame eyebrows by brushing them upwards with an eyebrow mousse or clear mascara.

Perfect your pluck

If the last time you tried to pluck your eyebrows you ended up with lop-sided ones or brows which made you look permanently surprised, go to a beautician, who will create the perfect shape by either plucking or waxing them, or by using a method known as 'threading'. Once the initial shape has been determined you can easily maintain it at home. • To avoid painful plucking, first numb the area to be plucked with a little clove oil or, make-up artists' favourite, baby's teething gel. • With the exception of the odd stray hair, always pluck from underneath the eyebrow. Hold the skin taut with one hand and pluck with the other, creating an arch from the point where your iris begins.

Magic up chiselled cheekbones

You can't alter the basic bone structure of your face, but you can achieve more prominent cheekbones with contouring and regular facial exercises (see Eva Fraser's work out on page 106).

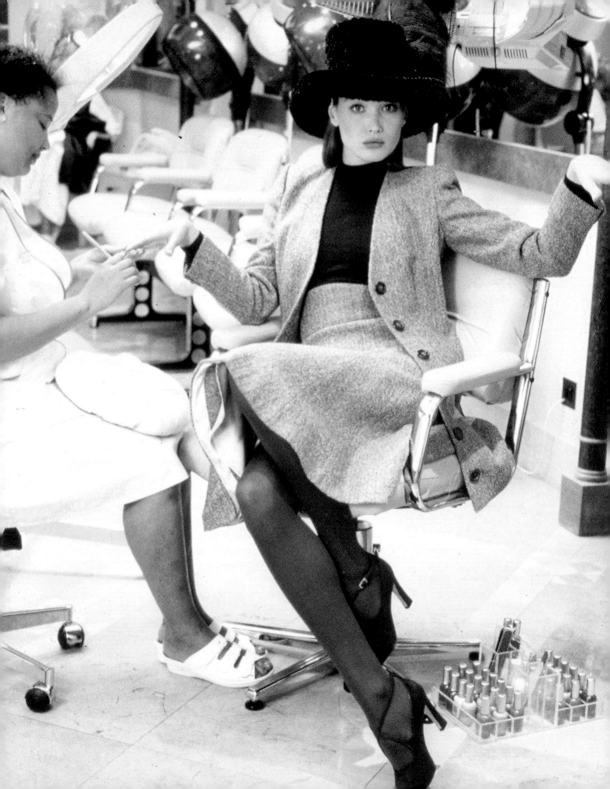

- To contour your face with make-up, Ruby suggests the following: Step one – Sweep ivory eyeshadow or highlighter across the top of the cheekbones. Step two – Add a wash of blush to the apple of your cheeks, sweeping upwards and outwards. Step three – Follow with a hint of colour just underneath the cheekbone. Blend.

Lip service

For an á la Julia Roberts smoulder, or to correct the shape of your lips, Ruby's trick is as follows: 'Taking a brush, draw a line around your lips with a pale foundation. Blend this into the lips before reshaping them with lip colour (also use a brush)'. • When applying lip colour, remember that paler colours illuminate and make lips appear bigger, while darker colours have a receding effect. • To achieve fuller lips without using make-up, plump them up by applying balm and then scrubbing them with a toothbrush, or try a special lip-plump product, such as Guerlain's Lip Lift or BeneFits' Lip Plump.

Give yourself an instant face-lift

If you have long hair, tying it back into a chignon or ponytail between the nape of your neck and crown of your head will lift your face. • A non-surgical face-lift, such as an electronic facial like C.A.C.I., can temporarily lift your face by using microcurrents. • For an instant lift, use one of the many face-lifts-in-a-jar – face masks and serums that temporarily firm the skin. Try Chanel's Firming Mask, YSL's Instant Firming Gel or Sisely's Tensor Immediate Lift.

Boost complexion

When your skin is crying out for nourishment, step up your skincare routine by using a serum daily before your moisturiser and a rehydrating mask twice weekly. • Brighten a dull complexion by sloughing off dead skin either with an exfoliant or by rubbing your face briskly with a face cloth. • Rehydrate your body from the inside by drinking two litres of purified or mineral water a day. • Rev up your circulation by massaging your face for a couple of minutes. • For an instant glow, splash your face with cold water before dusting blush to apples of cheeks.

Banish wrinkles

Temporarily plump up wrinkle-prone zones with anti-wrinkle miracle pads, patches or on-the-spot line-erasing lotions, such as La Prairie's Age-smoothing Concentrate, Prescriptives' Line, Spot, Wrinkle Retinol Repair or BeneFits' It Stick – a white liner to fill in wrinkles. • Ease facial tension by relaxing your muscles – this will also prevent lines appearing. • Eliminate frown lines by applying derma patches (known as 'frownies') to hold the muscles in place overnight. • Soften lines by massaging your face twice daily.

FASHION OVERHAUL

Style metamorphosis

No make-over is complete without a clothes revamp, and no other aspect of a make-over can make such a big impact on your image. But you don't have to wait until you get the chance to take part in a magazine or TV make-over, you can set about transforming yourself. • Buy a few magazines, earmark the looks that you like, and then set aside a day to visit shops and investigate creating a similar look, but one that is still individual to you (see page 67 for more tips on style). • If you just can't get it right yourself, visit an image consultant (also known as a wardrobe editor or stylist); many large stores now offer the service for free if you make a purchase.

Revamp your wardrobe

Take a good look at each and every item of clothing that you possess. Ask yourself 'Does it flatter me?' Decide how you could transform a garment by teaming it with something different, and consider what you need to give it that modern touch. • Think about colour: hold each item close to your face and see what it does for you. Throw out any hard-to-wear hues, unless these garments are to be worn below the waist. • Edit your wardrobe. Be ruthless: if it contains any clothes that you are really never going to wear again, donate them to a charity shop or jumble sale. • Revamp last year's fashions or inexpensive clothes either by teaming them with a strong accessory, or with striking, up-to-the-minute shoes.

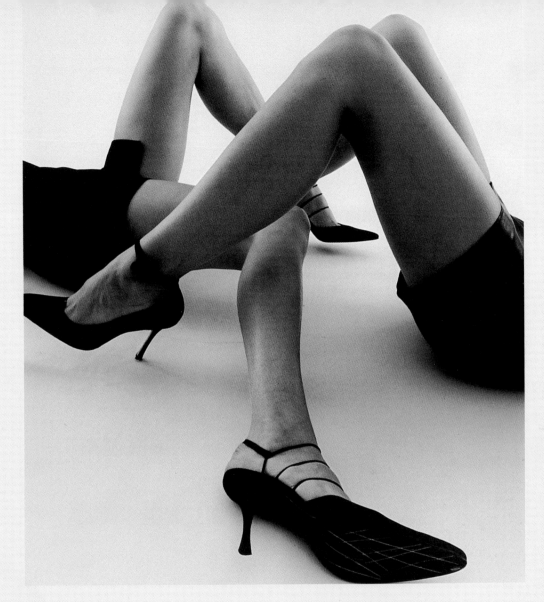

BODY REVAMP

Get a golden glow

Even out a blotchy skin tone or add just a hint of colour with fake tan. Exfoliate first, then apply body lotion before smoothing on a thin layer of self-tanning product. If it's more of a sun-kissed look you're after, apply two layers (see page 132 for self-tanning tips).

Create long, shapely legs

To give the illusion of longer legs, wear high heels. • Trousers that hang over your shoes or boots will also elongate your legs. • Shapely legs can be yours by walking up several flights of stairs each day or by working out on a Stairmaster. • For lean legs, don a pair of leg-slimming tights; these make legs appear toned by holding in any lumps and bumps.

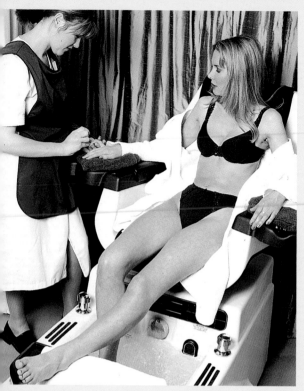

the affected areas. • When showering, aim the shower head on to the cellulite, interspersing cold water with hot, to disperse fatty deposits.

Firm up your butt

For a smoother, firmer bottom, shape up with simple bottom clenches. Clench buttocks, hold for a couple of seconds, then release; repeat a hundred times. Do this every day and witness the difference in just a few weeks. • To lift a droopy bottom instantly, cheat by wearing bottom-raising knickers. • If you are lacking in the shapely-bottom department, fill it out by wearing a pair of specially-designed padded panties.

Help your hands

Before you retire to bed, treat your mitts to a rehydrating face mask, cover them with cotton gloves and you'll have silky, soft hands by the morning. • Exfoliate your hands with a little blob of your face or body scrub. • Smother on hand cream at least twice a day (see page 134).

Neaten your nails

Paint your nails with a clear or coloured varnish or decorate them with nail art. • For instant shine without varnish, buff your nails using both sides of a nail buffer. • For a well-groomed set of nails, Gronya Logan, the Aveda Urban Retreat's head of beauty's tips are: 'Have regular manicures: they will improve the condition of your nails. To give your nails a new look, file them down to a two-millimetre edge, following the shape of your cuticle and squaring off slightly.'

REINVENT YOUR HAIR

Hair transformation

Hair is your strongest visual characteristic and changing it is one of the best ways to transform yourself from boring to bombshell. According to Antoinette Beenders, the Aveda Urban Retreat's creative director for hair: 'A new haircut can update you, make you look sexier, younger, smarter or more sophisticated'. Here are some ideas for changing your look. • Wearing your hair up, or pinning front sections back, are quick and easy ways in which to change your look. • Have

It's my turn – here I am at the Aveda Urban Retreat (frequented by the likes of Cher, Liz Hurley and Minnie Driver) having my own make-over.

Beautify your bust

Models make their breasts appear bigger by the clever use of cleavage-enhancing or breast-boosting bras and make-up. • Sweep bronzing powder across the curve of each breast, then smooth on body shimmer. • Firm up your bust with simple daily exercises. Clasp your hands together in front of your chest and push the palms together; repeat fifty times. • Invest in a good bra that not only lifts your breasts but also flatters your shape.

Combat cellulite

Combating cellulite requires a three-pronged attack: a healthy diet, exercise and home treatments. There follows a taster of the treatments that you can carry out at home (see page 130 for more tips). • Skin-brush stubborn zones daily. • Massage anti-cellulite cream into a versatile cut that you can wear in different ways. • If you have sleek, straight hair, you could try changing to a side, centre or zig-zag parting. • Revamp your hairstyle by adding lift at the roots. • Instead of wearing your hair forward, smooth it back off your face. • If you have short hair, gel or wax it back into a sleek finish (see Catwalk-style hair for more ideas on page 94).

Become colourful

Colouring your hair can have a huge impact on your image. Even going just a couple of shades lighter or darker, introducing colour around the face, or adding interesting high- or lowlights will give you a new look (see page 88). For instant colour, try colour mousses, colour-enhancing shampoos, conditioners and hair mascaras, or simply clip on coloured hairpieces.

Just-stepped-out-of-the-salon-looking hair

For salon-style volume, bounce and shine, utilise the excellent salon formula styling products (professional hair products or stylists' own product lines) on the market. • Invest in a hairdryer with the maximum number of heat and speed settings. • Equip yourself with the right tools: good brushes; Velcro rollers in different sizes; bendy sticks; heated appliances, such as straightening irons and heated rollers. • A shiny, sleek finish can be yours by applying an anti-frizz product or shine serum and then spritzing your hair with a gentle holding spray.

FINAL TOUCHES

Get sexy

Smooth, silky skin is sexy. To achieve this, exfoliate and skin brush daily, and wash the softness back into your skin by using a moisturising body wash followed by body lotion. • A seductive pout can be yours by drawing just outside the lip line of your Cupid's bow with a lip pencil, filling in lips with colour and adding a dab of gloss to the bottom lip. • Hair that is supershiny and cut in a feminine style that falls seductively across the face is deeply sexy. • To walk more provocatively, slightly exaggerate your wiggle. • In order to dress for ultimate sex

appeal, opt for highish heels, invest in a push-up bra and wear figure-skimming (but not clingy) clothes (see page 187 for more tips).

Grow inches taller

Wearing your hair in a high ponytail will give you instant height. • Correcting your stance can make you appear taller. In fact, if you practice The Alexander Technique, a postural discipline which re-educates you to stand correctly, you can add as much as an inch to your height. • High heels undoubtedly add inches, but avoid the break-neck stiletto types as they look too obvious. • Wearing the same colour from head to toe gives the illusion of height.

Sashay like a supermodel

To appear instantly more attractive, check your posture: lift your body from the chest and walk tall. • Shoes with a heel will help you to carry yourself like a model. • Now for the walk: imagine that you are walking along a chalked line, all the while keeping your body aligned with it. Swing your hips, but only a little mind or you will lose any model grace that you might possess.

Change your name

If you really want to go the whole hog in reinventing yourself, there's nothing like a great-sounding name to get you noticed. Elton John beats Reg Dwight, while Norma Jean doesn't quite have the same ring to it as Marilyn Monroe.

Revolutionise your smile

Remove unsightly stains and brighten your teeth by brushing them with a whitening toothpaste, such as Rembrant or Pearls. • Whiten discoloured teeth by having them bleached, and have any metal fillings replaced with white ones. • Have your teeth regularly cleaned and polished by a dentist. • Flesh-coloured, brownish- or terracotta-hued lipsticks make teeth look whiter.

Improve your voice

Speak clearly and confidently. • Inject enthusiasm into the tone of your voice rather than talking in a dull drone.

FAKING IT

Why not transform yourself with the help of a few tricks of the trade? I'm not talking about having to face the surgeon's knife, but clever little beauty-enhancing accoutrements. Here's the low-down on the latest innovations, together with some of the beauty industry's best-kept secrets.

Clip on, stick on or slip into a 'miracle' beauty aid and, in the nick of time, you'll have fluttering eyelashes, slimmer legs or a cleavage to die for. Don't worry about cheating nature: ask yourself how many people today are a hundred per cent 'natural'. Indeed, nearly every woman has coloured her hair or applied some sort of 'fake reality'; if she hasn't, she's simply missing out. So think of your false lashes or control knickers as tricks of the trade, not guilty secrets. In any case, these *faux* beauty innovations are fast becoming convincingly natural-looking, so who's to know that you're cheating anyway!

Let's start with your crowning glory and work down. Instead of being stuck with the short hair that you hate and having to suffer that laborious growing-out period, consider **hair extensions**. Perhaps your long tresses lack body and fullness? A few strategically placed extensions will add volume nicely. For an instant change, **hairpieces**, **wigs** and **false bangs** make great party numbers (see Naomi's hair piece, right).

Now on to your face. Have you ever wished that you could find some **magic potion** that would make your under-eye bags and wrinkles vanish miraculously? Well, I'll let you into a movie-business secret: movie stars including Marilyn Monroe used haemorrhoid cream to do just that. Before you wrinkle your nose in disgust, such new generation products as Irene Gail's Line-free Eyes and Eyesential – which temporarily

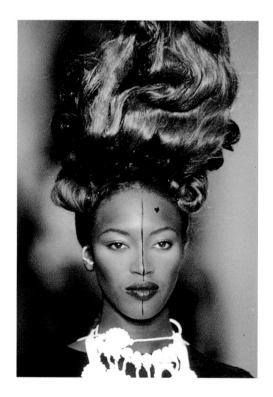

smooth out lines and banish bags – have been developed especially for the face without a haemorrhoid in sight! The line-free effect lasts for several hours and can be washed off at any stage. But take care to not move an inch for the few seconds while the potion is setting, or you will end up with more lines than you started with.

Having waged war on your wrinkles, it's now time to thicken, lengthen and fill out that sparse stubble that you call eyelashes with a few **false lashes**. The latest, individual lashes stay put, which means that there's no risk of one landing in your drink! Add one or two, or a little cluster of them to the outer corner of your upper eyelids. For serious fakers – and all those who are unhappy with their eye colour – you *can* have those dazzling-green or deep-pool-blue eyes you've always yearned for: purchase either tinted disposable **contact lenses** or the type that you simply remove at night.

If you want to wake up without having to look bare-faced or free of make-up splodges all over the pillow, the latest advanced techniques in **semi-permanent make-up** mean that you can have naturally rosy lips, a fuller-looking lash line and more defined eyebrows that stay that way for up to five years. Using coloured pigments, this form of tattooing requires several treatments, which allows for a gradual build-up. If you don't like the results, a good therapist should be equipped with a solution that removes the pigment.

How about an instant face-lift? If you really want to cheat, do what cover girls do to create that uplifted look and **tape** your face back at the hairline with micropore tape (found at most pharmacies) or such purpose-made tapes as Mark Trainers' Miracle Lift Tape.

If you weren't lucky enough to be born with a Cindy Crawford beauty spot, you can add a sensual **beauty mark** yourself by either drawing one with a brown eyeliner pencil, or applying one of the stick-on types from a beauty-mark kit such as Temptu's.

Moving swiftly on to your body: if your bust resembles little more than bee stings, try slipping a pair of breast-enhancing **gel pads** into your bra. If you don't want to run the risk of having what others thought were your god-given boobs land on the dance floor, shop around for a **booster bra**, such as the Magic Bra, which comes ready-stuffed with gel pads. If you want to go braless, a good trick for creating pert breasts is to stick tape underneath them or to use purpose-made

sticky pads. For those who are well endowed yet still lack a pneumatic, Pamela Anderson-style cleavage, invest in a cleavage-enhancing **push-up bra**, such as the Wonderbra.

Talking of pushing up, perhaps gravity is pulling your bottom a little too far south. If so, try **bottom-sculpting knickers** for a derrière to be proud of. Remaining on the underwear front, there are also **control knickers** that will give you a nipped-in waist while simultaneously flattening your tummy with their reinforced panels. Legs can be moulded into shape with **slimming tights** (and there's an added bonus: allegedly they improve circulation and reduce cellulite, too).

Turn yourself into an art form with **body art** (see picture below). A tattoo is too permanent a

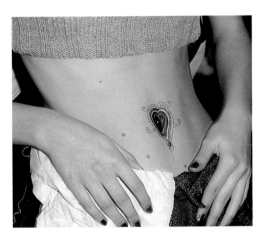

form of body art for most people, but you can now opt for more temporary designs using henna and found in the DIY kits available.

If there's one area with which most of us need a helping hand it's our nails. The tips of chewed, chipped or weak nails can be built up with a fibrous or acrylic substance or, if you prefer, you can still buy the stick-on nail. **Shaped-adhesive nail covers** will do away with the messy process of applying polish altogether.

Now don't go thinking that you can buy all these ingenious beauty innovations and then rest on your laurels. Work at looking after yourself or your partner will be in for a terrific shock when he or she sees you minus all your beauty aids!

CREATE YOUR OWN PERSONAL BEAUTY STYLE

We all have physical attributes that we can cultivate. Here's how to maximise your positive points, play down your bad ones, turn your flaws into assets and create your own beauty trademark.

CREATE YOUR INDIVIDUAL BEAUTY TRADEMARK

A modern beauty imperative is to flaunt some novel feature that makes you stand out from the crowd. It could be anything from the offbeat to the low-key: but it's often the subtle changes that create the most impact. Nails are a mainstay beauty feature; paint them in a show-off shade, alternate the colours on each nail by using two or three different polishes, or decorate each with a flower or rhinestone. Hair is another useful tool: with colour, styling or, if it's long, by adding accessories, your crowning glory can be transformed into an alluring trademark. For that pursued-by-the-paparazzi look, don a pair of fancy sunglasses. Alternatively, wear an unusual piece of jewellery, such as a choker or toe-ring.

From *mehndi* flowers for navels to face jewels, bindi dots, henna bracelets or little motifs for ankles, a great way of adding a stamp of individuality is to decorate a part of your body with elaborate body art. With Demi Moore, Madonna, Daryl Hanner, Sophie Dahl and many other celebrities sporting body art, it has become very *à la mode*. Create your own design or follow a pattern by using one of the temporary DIY kits which last several weeks, such as Temptu's Ceremonial Body Art, Revlon's Street-wear Art Pencil and Tattoo Sealer or Urban Decay's Body Art Kit.

DISCOVER YOUR BEAUTY TRAIT

Beauty demands that you be yourself and express your individuality, so start by looking for a beauty trait that makes you both unique and striking. If it's not obvious to you, ask your friends and partner. Study other people, as well as pictures of actresses and models, to try to identify what makes them special.

Here are a few suggestions regarding the characteristics that could become your personal beauty trait: a strong or delicate bone structure, your hair, smile, skin tone, a prominent or unusually shaped nose, long neck, a mole, freckles, large mouth, small lips, big eyes, deep-set eyes, hooded eyes, sparse or heavy eyebrows, a dimple.

You only have to glance at magazines to see how dozens of celebrities have made a beauty trait of a striking feature or even a so-called 'imperfection': think of Brook Shields' heavy eyebrows; Belinda Carlisle's dimples; Lauren Hutton's gap between her teeth; Barbra Steisand, Angelica Huston and Sandra Bullock's strong noses; Cindy Crawford's mole; Charlotte Rampling's hooded eyes; and Sigourney Weaver and Holly Hunter's thin lips.

Whether it's your most prized feature or a so-called 'flaw', make this characteristic a focal point and, wherever possible (you cannot exactly highlight a dimple), draw attention to it by playing it up, highlighting or defining it.

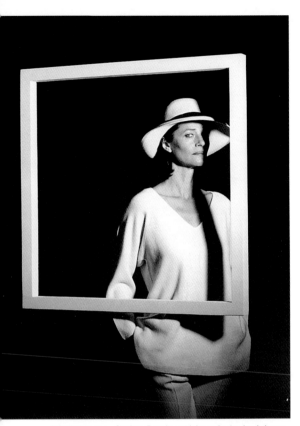

Individual beauty – Charlotte Rampling with her seductive, hooded eyes.

TURN YOUR FLAWS INTO ASSETS

If you are unhappy with a particular feature you could always resort to the scalpel, of course, but surgery might take away the very thing that makes you special.

It's not only classically pretty or perfectly formed features that give a face individual beauty style. In fact, you might find that it is precisely the feature that you detest the most (such as a prominent nose or a mole), that becomes your USP (unique selling point). Besides, what you regard as a flaw others may look upon as a plus point. For most of my teenage years I hated my large, 'blubbery' lips and consequently got through pots of concealer in trying to make them appear smaller. Then Julia Roberts appeared on the scene and I wished mine were even bigger!

PLAY DOWN YOUR BAD POINTS

Here are some easy solutions for drawing attention away from problem features.

Sticking-out ears: a sensuous mouth or dazzling smile will divert attention away from sticking-out ears. Also, if your hair is long enough, you may want to wear it in such a way that it falls around the sides of your face.

A protruding chin: shift attention from your chin by having your hair cut in a style that softens rather than frames your jaw line. If your hair is long, wear it layered to avoid a witch-like appearance or tie it back for a regal look.

A receding hairline or high forehead: draw the emphasis away from your hairline by: highlighting your eyes; dusting soft, brown powder along the hairline; sweeping your hair back off your face, tying it back or wearing a fringe.

A bulbous nose: play up your eyes, brows, lips or cheekbones to distract the eye from your nose.

Wonky lips: correct these by taking a brush loaded with a little concealer or foundation and then drawing a line over the part of lip that needs adjusting, before applying lip colour.

A double chin: dust soft, brown powder over your excess chin.

High colour: tone down a red face by applying a green-tinted cosmetic primer, base or skin tint before using foundation.

Jowls: always hold your chin up – jowls are most noticeable when you tilt your head downwards. Highlighting your cheekbones and colouring your lips also draws attention away.

Harelip: also known as a cleft lip, this is where the top lip is split and turned up. Occasionally it can look sexy, but if this is not the case, wear neutral lip colours and play up your eye area.

Birthmarks: cover birthmarks with camouflage preparations like Dermablend and Keromask. As port-wine stains are pinkish-red in colour they are more tricky to conceal, so try a green-tinted primer beneath a camouflage product.

Vitiligo: vitiligo is a lack of pigment in certain areas, which results in patchy-looking skin. Even out the skin tone by darkening the white patches with camouflage products, long-lasting foundation or theatrical make-up.

BOBBI BROWN'S 'IMPERFECT' BEAUTY

Bobbi Brown is one of the world's top make-up artists. She has her own leading signature make-up range and is the author of a best-selling book, *Bobbi Brown Beauty* (HarperStyle, 1997), in which you will find chapters devoted to personal beauty style.

Bobbi believes that you can turn a physical flaw into your most striking feature. She has listed some such striking beauty traits here, together with more general beauty looks from which a woman can develop her own individual beauty style.

A strong nose: 'I find distinctive noses to be a regal and powerful element of beauty. It is one trait, however, that you may not like about yourself as a teenager but will surely grow into and love as an adult. Do not try to shade the nose or change it with make-up – that will only make your nose look like it is smudged with dirt.'

A round face: 'It is a mistake to try to sculpt in cheekbones with make-up. Instead, line your eyes or play with lip colours and rejoice in the knowledge that you will always have a young appearance thanks to your face shape. Models often have this trait, which is one of the reasons why they photograph so well.'

Deep-set eyes: 'Lining eyes with a fine, dark line is the best way to open deep-set eyes. Avoid dark colours on the lid – use light-to-medium shadows instead. Apply highlighter at the brow line.'

Small lips: 'Do not attempt to create a bigger mouth by pencil-lining beyond the edge of your mouth – it tends to look silly. Instead, use a lip pencil to define your mouth, going to the full extent of your natural lip line. Wear light-to-medium colours on your mouth and put the focus on your eyes.'

'Bedroom' or hooded eyes: 'Women complain about hooded eyes all the time. I find them to be sexy and mysterious. Do not use dark shadow on the lid in an attempt to make your eyes stand out more – that will only blacken and further recess them. Instead, line your eyes with a stroke wide enough still to be visible when your eyes are open. A slight contour to eyes with light/medium shadow is a good technique to try. And don't forget to use a well-shaped brow to achieve good overall eye definition.'

Pale skin: 'So many women with pale skin search for the perfect bronzing powder; instead, just make yourself as pale and soft as you can. Never go into the sun.'

Big brows: 'Don't be tempted to change your brow shape since a weighty eyebrow probably complements your features and frame. Instead, work on better defining your eyebrows. Pluck away any hairs between the brows and brush brow hairs up (using a firm toothbrush). If brows are sparse in spots, fill in using a shadow and brow brush.'

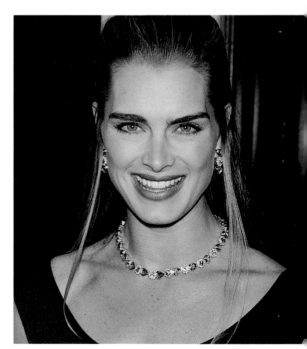

Brooke Shields's big brows are her beauty trademark.

CREATE THE PERFECT SILHOUETTE

Having focused on your facial features, now it is time to shift the attention to your figure by resolving to emphasise your plus points and disguise any body blips with the right clothing.

A fuller figure? Don't hide your body under big, chunky or bulky clothes – they may be comfy, but they'll add extra inches to your size. Desperately trying to squeeze your bulges into the pencil skirt that you wore when you were a size 12 is also a no-no, unless you want to emphasise your blubbery bits. Opt for tailored, figure-skimming clothes in fluid fabrics, rather than clingy garments. Jackets are slimming; single-breasted more so than double-breasted. Colour-wise, dark shades recede and will streamline your figure, yet don't overlook eye-catching hues and bold prints as these often look so striking they actually detract from your size. Chunky jewellery looks better on fuller figures than delicate pieces.

A pear-shaped figure? The classic pear-shaped figure is slim on top and a couple of dress sizes bigger around the bottom and hips. The trick is therefore to build up the top half and slim down the hips with streamlined trousers and skirts. Team trousers with a tunic-style top, long-length jacket or loose shirt that falls below your widest part. Steer clear of fitted dresses and clingy tops that have soft shoulders, and plump for clothes with a stronger shoulder line. But unless you want to look like a 1980s' power-dresser, choose garments with small shoulder pads.

Too busty? Show a little cleavage and wear plunging necklines by all means, but avoid clingy tops. You'll find that V-necks and cowl necks are generally more flattering than a round or high neckline. Fitted jackets and tops work better than their looser counterparts, as the latter tend to make busty women look 'mumsy'. Forget fussy tops with pockets, or blouses with frilly bits, as these draw attention to your bust.

Too small breasts? Give the impression that you have bigger breasts by wearing a push-up bra or breast-boosting bra complete with gel pads. And remember that you have one strong advantage over your bigger-busted sisters: you can go braless and wear those sexy slip dresses, low-backed numbers and fashionable sheers without your breasts hanging down to your waist!

Heavy legs? Clothes that accentuate heavy thighs include skirts that stop on the largest part of the thighs, waist-length tops and jackets, as well as tight, leggings-style trousers. When shopping for trousers, either streamline, boot-cut trousers that flare out very slightly at the hem, or straight-legged trousers are best, as they will slim down and lengthen the appearance of your legs. Matching your shoes and hoisery to your skirt colour also has a slimming effect.

Too petite? Give floor-sweeping clothes a miss: maxi-skirts and ankle-length coats will swamp you and will make you look even shorter. You may be tempted to wear very high heels, assuming that they will make up for your missing inches, but be aware that these could draw attention to your lack of height, especially if you teeter all over the place in a pair of break-neck stilettos.

A big bottom? The trick is to de-emphasise your hips and bottom, so avoid belts and waistbands that nip in the waist or you could end up by making your derrière look even larger. A-line skirts, shift dresses and waist-skimming clothes are more forgiving. Steer clear of any items that flare out from the hips; cropped jackets and tops that finish at the waist will also overemphasise less than slim hips or a big posterior. On the trouser front, the high-waisted styles with zips at the side or back flatter a big bottom, but avoid trousers that taper in at the ankle, opting for the straight-legged or boot-cut types instead.

A podgy stomach? Tight-fitting tops, and dresses and skirts with gathers or pleats will highlight a podgy stomach, whereas waistless shifts, tunic-style tops and long-length jackets appear to knock off pounds. Refrain also from wearing tight, bias-cut or pencil skirts and clingy, leggings-style trousers.

BEAUTY IN A FLASH

We all want to look great, but today's hectic lifestyles mean that few of us have hours to spend on pampering our bodies to perfection. With the following short cuts to looking good, even the busiest high-flyer will be able to squeeze a few beauty enhancers into her hectic schedule and look fabulous in a matter of minutes.

LABOUR-SAVING LOCKS

Washing, styling, blow-drying – not to mention lengthy visits to the hairdresser's – are high on the list of time-consumers. So how can you crack the art of having great looking hair with minimum effort? For starters, hair that is cut well will fall into shape effortlessly, so save time on upkeep by finding a good hairdresser. Choose a natural-looking, low-maintenance style that works with your hair's texture and doesn't need too much taming with hairdryers and heated appliances. You could always try a shampoo that helps speed up the drying process, such as JF Lazartigue's Rapid Drying Shampoo. If you have poker-straight hair, a blunt cut or bob will be easy to style, while for slightly wavy locks or curly hair, a layered, tousled look that you can run your hands through and leave to dry naturally is ideal; trying to straighten curly hair or *vice versa* will cost you precious time.

Styling in a hurry

If you have short hair, all it takes is a squirt of sculpting lotion, gel or mousse and you can leave your locks to dry naturally. The long haired should use styling products that smooth, straighten and add thickness and shine, which will cut down on blow-drying time because they do the styling work for you. Try VO5's 3-in-1 Styler, Nicky Clarke's Hairomatherapy Lift, Thicken and Shine Spray or Sebastian's Gelée Performance Active Conditioner and Styling Gel. To save time on styling, wind hair in rollers and allow to set while you do your make-up.

Wash 'n' go

Very few of us have time to hang around the bathroom 'drip-drying' while our conditioner works. Yet you shouldn't skip this essential step if you want beautiful hair. If you have short hair, you can get away with using a combined shampoo and conditioner, such as L'Oréal's Elvive Revitalising 2-in-1 or Vidal Sassoon's Wash 'n' Go. Those with long or damaged hair can opt for a good leave-in conditioner: try Inne's Strengthening Extract, Aveda's Elixir or Pantene's Intensive Leave-in Strengthening Serum. Hair treatments don't have to be exclusively for ladies of leisure: you can just pop on an intensive hair mask, such as Phytologie's Phytomoelle Overnight Mask, before you retire to bed and let it do the work while you sleep.

Low-maintenance colour

You can't escape the fact that colouring hair is a high-maintenance procedure. Before embarking on having your hair coloured, remember that the further away from your natural shade the colour is, the more frequent the upkeep. To cut down on visits to the salon, try these tips. Touch up regrowth or grey hairs with a colour wand like Dior's Mascara Flash for Hair, which comes in seventeen shades, or Trevor Sorbie's Highliter Wand. Sprinkle a little dry shampoo or talc on your roots to defuse the darkness of root growth. Enrich colour that has faded with a colour-enhancing shampoo or conditioner, such as Aveda's colour shampoos and conditioners.

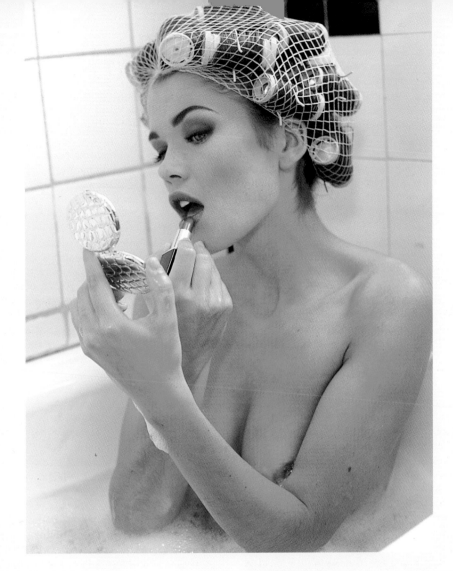

No time to shampoo

You've been asked out to a fancy restaurant but haven't got the usual half-hour that it takes to wash, dry and style your hair. Don't panic: for freshly-washed-looking hair in a flash, try the following. If your hair is greasy, sprinkle on a little dry shampoo or talcum powder at the roots and brush through. To put style and volume back into your hair, spritz it with a styling lotion, turn your head upside down and blast with a hairdryer. Alternatively, disguise grease or dirt by smothering your hair with wax, gel or pomade, such as Kiehl's Wet-look Groomer or Oribe's Pomade, before slicking your hair back with a comb or, if your hair is long, scraping it up into a ponytail or twisting it into a chignon and securing with a slide. For that totally clean feeling, you need to freshen up the smell of your hair. Spray your favourite scent or toner into the air and walk through the perfumed mist, or try hair-freshening sprays, such as L'Occitane's Purifying Spray For Hair or Kenzo's Perfumed Hair Mist.

Nippy nails

Keep your nails well trimmed and they will look groomed without the need to spend time or money on a manicure. For shiny nails minus the hassle of applying varnish, simply buff with a nail buffer. If you don't dare to go naked, opt for a fast-drying varnish, such as Revlon's Top Speed Enamel, Maybelline's Express Finish Nail Polish or Rimmel's 60 Second Nail Polish. Alternatively, speed up drying times with a spray, like Sally Hanson's Dry Fast Nail Spray or Opi's Rapidry Spray, and use Sally Hanson's Manicure Clean Up Stick to magic away any mistakes. Retouching is a bind, so remember that using a light shade makes this easier. To avoid having to revarnish too often try Max Factor's Diamond Hard, Helena Rubinstein's Long-lasting Varnish or Givenchy's Long Lasting Glossy Nail Colour. Put an end to chipping polish with peel-off formulas, such as Lancôme's Vernis Zapping Peel Off Varnish. Rather than having to muck around applying a base, second and top coat, choose a one-coat varnish like Cover Girl's 3-in-1 Nail Sticks or Sally Hanson's One Coat.

MAKE-UP SHORT CUTS

Are you guilty of applying make-up on the bus or train? Stop this bad beauty habit and, instead, cut down on make-up-application time with these time-savers. Cosmetic companies have helped you to cut corners and saved you from carrying around a hefty bag laden with dozens of cosmetics by cleverly devising multi-purpose products that can be used on the lips, cheeks and eyes. Try Virgin Vie's All Rounder, Colourings' Complete Colour, BeneFit's Nine One One wand, Trucco's Lip and Face Compact, Bobbi Brown's Bronzing Stick, Aveda's One Colour Plus Uruka, Nars' The Multiple or Vincent Longo's Lip/Eye Pencil.

Long-lasting make-up means that you don't have to waste time retouching as lipstick, foundation and eyeshadow stays put – even when eating or kissing. Do away with make-up application altogether by investing in semi-permanent make-up, such as eyeliner, brow-shading and lip colour that lasts for five years.

Base in a jiffy

To save on time-intensive application, try a multi-purpose base, such as YSL's 4-in-1 Sheer Powder Crème Veil, Max Factor's 3-in-1 Complete Coverage Make-up, Virgin Vie's One Step Face Base, Estée Lauder's Minute Make-up or Stila's Complete Coverage Make-up. Another option is to use a dab of base or concealer only where you need it. For long-lasting results, try L'Oréal's Colour Endure Foundation, Versace's Long-lasting Hydrating Foundation, Dior's Long-wearing Hydrating Concealer or Revlon's ColorStay Foundation. If you haven't got time to apply a base, one application of fake tan will give your skin a touch of colour and warmth that lasts for several days.

Swift blush

Imparting a rosy glow to your cheeks is quick and easy to achieve: if you wear nothing but blush on your skin, a cream, gel or stain blush can be applied swiftly to naked skin (powder blush only really sits well on a foundation or powder base). If you only want to carry the bare essentials in your hand bag, for retouching, both a multipurpose product or a little lipstick smoothed on cheeks can also be used as blush.

One-minute eyes

Do away with lengthy mascara applications by tinting your eyelashes with a home eyelash-dye kit or by having them dyed professionally at a salon. You can also darken brows; the effect should last for up to a month. If you prefer the stronger and longer-lasting effect of liquid eyeliners to pencils, opt for fool-proof liner pens, such as Lancôme's Artliner or Maybelline's Liner Express. Wave goodbye to endless retouching by finding a good, long-lasting eyeshadow, such as Clinique's Stay The Day or Avon's Perfect Wear. Instead of using different products on your eyes and brows, use one product for both features. For example, brown eyeshadow works as an eyeliner and a brow-definer, while your mascara can even double up to thicken and darken brows. Another option is dual-purpose products, such as Elizabeth Arden's Dual Perfection Brow Shaper and Eyeliner.

Lasting lip colour

Lipstick can be fiddly to apply, so for extra-fast results just add a slick of coloured gloss: try Almay's Lip Balm With Colour, MAC's Lip Glass, Blistex's Lip Tone or Stila's Lip Gloss. For lipstick that stays the day use Cover Girl's Continuous Colour Self-renewing Lipstick, Revlon's MoistureStay or Dior's Diorific Long-wearing Lipstick. You can also try a self-renewing lipstick, such as Max Factor's Lasting Colour Self Renew Lipstick, that refreshes itself when you press your lips together. Cut down on application time by using a lipstick and liner in one. Plump for products like Elizabeth Arden's Exceptional Lip Talkers or Maybelline's Lip Express.

LOW MAINTAINANCE SKIN AND BODYCARE

To achieve a smooth, silky skin with minimum effort, incorporate exfoliation into your daily ablutions by using a dual-purpose shower gel and exfoliant, such as Revlon's Dry Skin Relief Intensive Exfoliating Shower Gel; or try a conditioning shower gel, such as Oil of Ulay's Moisturising Body Wash, Johnson's PH 5.5 2-in-1 Shower Gel and Body Moisturiser or St Ives' Formula Cocoa Butter Moisturising Body Wash. While your deodorant is drying, a faster alternative to body cream is a spray-on lotion like Lancôme's Resource Drenching Body Spray or Palmer's Aloe Vera Formula Body Spray.

Whether you wax or shave, this beauty headache can be cut out completely by having excess hair permanently removed by laser or electrolysis. If the drying time puts you off fake tan, experiment with one of the fast-drying self-tans in spray form, such as Ecotan's Self Tan and La Prairie's Spray Self Tan. To cut corners on your body- and handcare, as well as your skincare, use all-encompassing, multi-purpose creams and lotions that can be used on your face, body, hands, any dry patches, cuticles and feet; some of these include L'Occitane's Shea Butter Cold Cream and Nivea's All Soft Intensive Moisturising Cream for both body and face.

Skincare short cuts

Keep your skincare regime pared down by choosing a product that cleanses and tones in one step: try Elizabeth Arden's 2-in-1 Cleanser and Toner, Vichy's One-step Cleanse, RoC's 2-in-1 Cleanser and Freshener for Face and Eyes or Synergie's Refreshing 2-in-1 Gentle Cleanser and Toner. Alternatively, perform your own simultaneous cleanse and tone by removing cleanser with a muslin cloth, then wetting the cloth and patting it onto your face. No time to hang around for twenty minutes while your face mask works? How about a flash balm or fast working mask, such as No 7's 3 Minute Energising Mask, Clarins' Beauty Flash Balm, Bioré's sixty-second Self-Heating Mask or Decleor's Instant Beauty Booster? For a nourishing boost, apply a moisturising mask or treatment before you go to bed, such as Guerlain's Issima Midnight Secret or La Formule's Night Shift. No low-maintenance beauty will have time for a full facial workout, but you can still keep some muscles taut by chewing gum (sugar-free, please!).

FITNESS IN A FLASH

For the busy high-flyer, joining a gym or attending a regular exercise class is totally out of the question. Therefore, the answer is to try home-exercising, as this cuts down on travelling time, not to mention cost, and can be squeezed in early morning or at night. Different ways of keeping fit at home include yoga, stretching exercises, working out in front of an exercise video, using home-exercise equipment or a simple resistance band (the latter is ideal for use both at home and when travelling).

For those who cannot commit to even twenty minutes of home-exercising, there are still ways of incorporating exercise into your daily life: run up escalators, walk up stairs instead of taking the lift and, when taking public transport, get off the train or bus a stop earlier and walk the remaining distance. When you are at home, do bottom clenches while washing up or cleaning your teeth, and sit-ups while watching TV.

LOOKING GOOD ON A SHOESTRING

We can't all afford to lavish money on luxury beauty products and designer clothes, but this doesn't mean that we have to look second-rate. Here are dozens of tips to help you to look good for less money.

• **Make your own** perfumed body lotion by adding a couple of drops of your favourite scent or essential oil to an unfragranced lotion.

• **Double up or triple** the use of items of your make-up. For example: use your lipstick as a blusher; your blusher as a lip colour and eyeshadow; your lip pencils as eye pencils; your eye pencils as lip and brow pencils; and your eyeshadow, liner and mascara as brow-definers.

Models **save on the cost of rollers** by winding their hair around a couple of empty soft-drink cans to straighten hair and add volume to the roots.

• Economise by purchasing **multi-purpose beauty products**, such as combined cleansers and toners; creams that can be used on the hands, lips, neck and décolletage; and cosmetics 'in one', such as a combined blusher, lipstick and eye colour.

• Rather than paying for a ready-made eye-bath solution, **bathe your eyes** in mineral water to freshen them up.

• To achieve model-like hair without the cost of visiting a salon, **invest in hair maestros' products**, many of which are surprisingly inexpensive. Sam McKnight, Frédéric Fekkai, John Frieda, Nicky Clarke, Charles Worthington and Oribe are just some of the stylists whose own ranges are sold in supermarkets, pharmacies and hair salons.

• **Decant inexpensive** skin- and bodycare products into attractive jars or empty pots from more costly cosmetic ranges. Psychologically, you will be lulled into thinking that you are using luxury products.

• Save money by **investing in all-season wear** – items of clothing that can be worn all year round – as well as in all-occasion wear that can be pared down for day and jazzed up for evening.

• Turn a rich moisturiser or night cream into a light day cream by **wetting your fingers** and mixing it in the palm of your hand, before applying it.

• Wiping a beetroot across your lips makes for a cheap, **natural lip stain**. Red or pink food colouring will also stain your lips for a fraction of the cost of a cosmetic stain.

- More and more cosmetics companies who advertise in the glossy women's magazines are giving away **samples of moisturisers**, cleansers and other products. Collect these sachets; they are the perfect size for weekends away.

- Toothpaste is not only good for teeth – it can double up as a **spot-zapper** and, if you've overdone it with the fake tan, rub on a little toothpaste and it will help fade the mistake.

- Raid your kitchen cupboard for **natural beauty solutions** (see page 164 for recipes).

- Rather than paying out for dumbbells, for a **cheap home workout**, use cans of beans, for example, or bags of sugar instead.

- **Cut-price and designer clothes** can be found at factory shops, discount-clothes stores and even some supermarkets. Less obvious bargain-hunting places include army-surplus stores, dancewear and sportswear shops.

- **Trade your old clothes** for new at a nearly-new shop, clothes agency or second-hand designer boutique.

- Instead of using expensive cuticle cream, rub **almond oil** into your nails to nourish them and soften your cuticles.

- If you can't afford your **favourite perfume**, you can still wear the fragrance in a less expensive form, such as a body spray, powder, shower gel or deodorant.

- **Save on mascara** by dyeing your eyelashes using a home eyelash-tint kit.

- To **freshen your face**, pour mineral water into a small atomiser or plant spray and spritz face.

- **Get a free make-over**. Most of the new-generation make-up stores and counters offer free make-overs in the hope that you will purchase some of their products. Unless stated, you are under no obligation to buy.

- Look out for the major **cosmetics houses' promotions**. Buy one or two products and you will qualify for all sorts of freebies, from a complimentary facial to a cosmetic bag.

- **Update your make-up** for free by mixing together different shades of your existing lipsticks or eyeshadows to create a palette of new colours.

- To make your expensive toner go further, **dilute with witch hazel** or rose-water.

- Save money by having a **cut without a blow-dry**; by the time the hairdresser has finished cutting your hair it will be almost dry.

> To make their own, **custom-made coloured lip gloss**, make-up artists mix a little crushed eyeshadow, blusher or lipstick with Vaseline Petroleum Jelly or lip balm.

- When you just can't squeeze any more cream out of a tube, **cut it in half** – you'll be surprised at how much is left inside.

- For a **cost-free toner**, wet a muslin cloth with cold water and cover your face with it for a few seconds. Alternatively, splash your face a couple of times with cold water.

- Make your own **massage oil** by adding a few drops of your favourite essential oil to a carrier oil, such as almond or olive oil.

- Ask at cosmetic counters for **trial-sized products**. They are a good way of testing if you like a product and are the perfect size to pop into your handbag or take on holiday. (The trick to getting freebie samples is to ask the beauty consultant for advice.)

- Save on **facial exfoliants** by rubbing your face with a dry towel before cleansing, or with a damp face cloth afterwards. Turn to page 164 for recipes for cheap home-made exfoliants.

- **Second-hand chic** can be found at charity shops, flea markets, thrift stores, jumble sales, antique shops and second-hand designer boutiques. Don't discard hand-me-downs: you might find that your mother's bouclé coat becomes your all-time favourite item.

- For a **cheap body scrub**, take a handful of finely-ground salt into the shower.

- Vaseline Petroleum Jelly makes a **good lip balm** and can also be used to groom your eyebrows.

- If you've run out of **shower gel**, a mild shampoo can double up as both.

- Instead of purchasing eye masks, place used, **chilled tea bags** over your eyes.

- For a **cheap spot lotion**, dab on lemon juice.

- Save your **old toothbrush**, this works well as both an eyebrow brush and a lip exfoliant.

- Cut down on cosmetics' costs by adding a tiny dollop of moisturiser to your foundation to turn it into a **tinted moisturiser**.

- If you want to try brightly coloured make-up or nail vanish experiment with **cheaper brands**, they often have the widest range of colours.

- For a **cost-free, temporary touch-up** coat the odd grey hair with your mascara.

- Save on buying foundation by using **fake tan**; one application will last two – three days.

- Several big-name designers have created **special collections** (ranges which cost considerably less then their main label designs). Buy them in high-street chains, department stores and mail-order catalogues. When shopping, look for the 'designed by' signs.

- Keep your eyebrows in place with a **slick of hairspray** gel or styling lotion (ensure that you spray it onto your hand first).

- If you are blonde and your hair has turned brassy in the sun, yet you can't afford a trip to the hairdresser's, **tone the colour down** temporarily with tomato ketchup. Smother your hair in the ketchup, leave it on for ten minutes and then wash it off.

> Save money by trawling through lingerie shops for **underwear that doubles up as outerwear**. A pure silk slip will cost a fraction of the price of an evening frock; dress it up with a stunning piece of jewellery and no one will know the difference.

- Use a rolling pin, small jar or pebble as a **foot-massager**. Place under the sole of your foot and massage using gentle movements.

- **Children's clothes** are generally less expensive than adults', and many child-sized T-shirts, cardigans and tank tops will fit slim grown-ups.

- Make your own **hair treatment** by warming up a little olive or almond oil. Apply to your hair before wrapping in warm towels and leaving for twenty minutes.

- **Lavender essential oil** (one of the less expensive aromatherapy oils) can be used for a multitude of purposes: to heal spots, help you sleep, revive your energy or, when diluted with water, as an underarm deodorant.

- Don't dismiss **supermarkets' own ranges** or mass market brands: often a great deal of research has gone into developing these products.

- Make your own **herbal teas** by steeping fresh herbs in an infuser.

- **A bowl of water** placed in a centrally-heated room will save you buying a humidifier.

- For a **cheap, fake, facial tan**, mix the spice turmeric with yoghurt (see page 165 for the full home-made recipe).

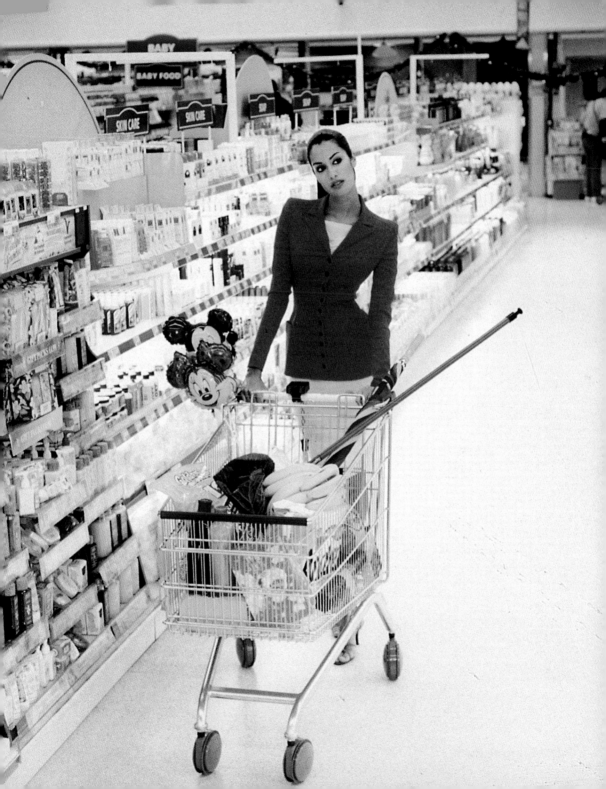

BEAUTY CRIMES

1 Don't go to bed with your make-up on

A little bit of lipstick isn't exactly a deadly poison that will cause a slow death of beauty in the night. But go to bed still wearing foundation or eye make-up, and you could end up in a real mess: the stale make-up will clog the pores and settle in lines, resulting in spots and wrinkles.

2 Never squeeze spots

Unless you have a pimple with such a ripe head on it that it is about to burst, don't attempt to squeeze. Picking aggravates the spot and, even if you are careful and use tissues, the bacteria could spread under the skin, producing more spots.

3 Forget sharing make-up

You may be itching to try out your best friend's up-to-the-minute, plum-coloured lip pencil, but if she suffers from cold sores you could end up catching this herpes virus, which tends to stick around for good. Sharing eye make-up is also a definite no-no: contagious eye infections like conjunctivitis can easily be spread through borrowing eyeliners, mascaras and eyeshadows.

4 No frowning, please

Many of us fall into this habit unknowingly, especially when we are working or studying hard. Unless you welcome frown lines, smooth out your forehead by opening your eyes wider whenever you feel a frown coming on.

5 Don't bite your nails

Chewed nails look unsightly and give the impression that you don't give a damn about your appearance. From the health aspect, not only can nibbling cause infection, but if you were to peer through a microscope at the zillions of bacteria happily nestling under your fingernails, it's unlikely that you'd ever nibble them again.

6 Fling out the soap

By using soap you are stripping your skin's acid mantle, leaving it dehydrated. Soap leaves behind a residue and also contains surfactants, which are irritants. If you like to wash your face rather than wipe it, use a cleansing bar: these look and feel like soap but are actually soap-free.

7 Refrain from touching your face

You've walked the dog, put the rubbish out and travelled to work; sitting at your desk you start playing with your face – rubbing your forehead and searching for any rough areas on your cheeks. As you transfer the morning's grime and germs from your fingers onto your face, you are simultaneously spreading infection, oil and bacteria, resulting in spots, dry patches and sensitive skin, so leave your face alone.

8 Avoid licking your lips

Whether you are licking your lips to achieve that sultry, wet-look pout, or are wetting them because it's a habit – stop! Carry on, and you'll end up with crusty, dehydrated lips. Just try applying lipstick to lips in this state.

9 Stop assaulting your hair

Pulling and fiddling with your hair can become a bad habit which damages the hair's cuticles, and could affect the hair follicle causing permanent hair loss. Scraping hair back into too tight a pony tail is another hair sin.

10 Don't slouch

You might be a dead ringer for Naomi Campbell, but if you stand with hunched shoulders, you may as well be Quasimodo. Poor posture destroys good looks and can lead to health problems, such as backache and indigestion.

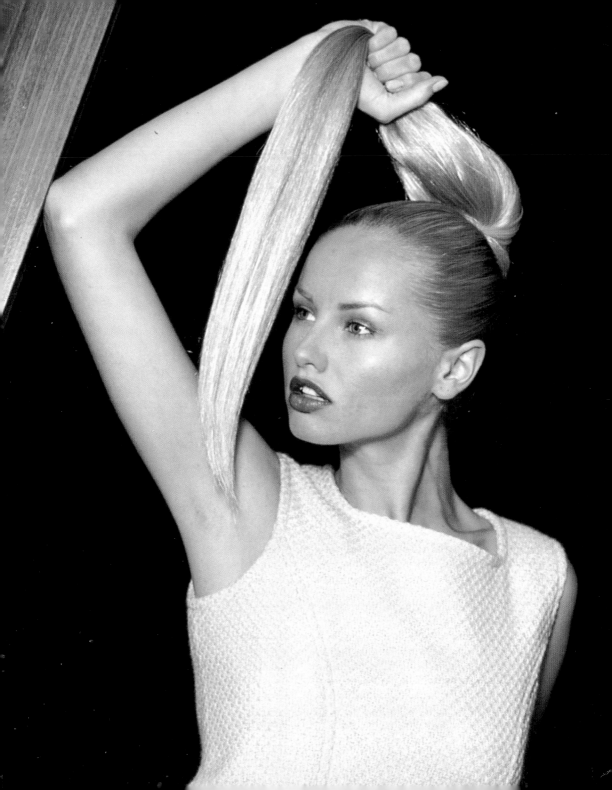

MALE MATTERS

There was a time when men used nothing
but carbolic soap and a splash of Old Spice.
Now they are raiding women's make-up bags
and are even painting their nails!

To all you men out there: let me reassure you that
it is no longer considered vain or effeminate to
care for your appearance. Anyway, you have
always been the vainer of the sexes: remember
the Greek legend of Narcissus? He became so
obsessed with his reflection in a pool that he
stared at it day in, day out, until the narcissistic
fool eventually died of starvation. Another vain
chap was Oscar Wilde's character Dorian Grey,
who made a diabolical pact to preserve his
looks. They may be fictional characters, but
there's a certain element of truth in their
behaviour – isn't there?

While women tend to look in a mirror and
criticise what they see, men typically smile
pleasingly at the image staring back at them.
Nonetheless, the growth in the male cosmetics
market is proof that men are dedicating more
time, money and effort to grooming. Having been
seduced by cosmetic ranges, men are now
showing up at beauty salons – not just for a
massage, but for facials, hair removal, eyelash
tints, manicures and even non-surgical face-lifts,
too. A few are even taking it a step further by
wearing nail polish, albeit in masculine shades

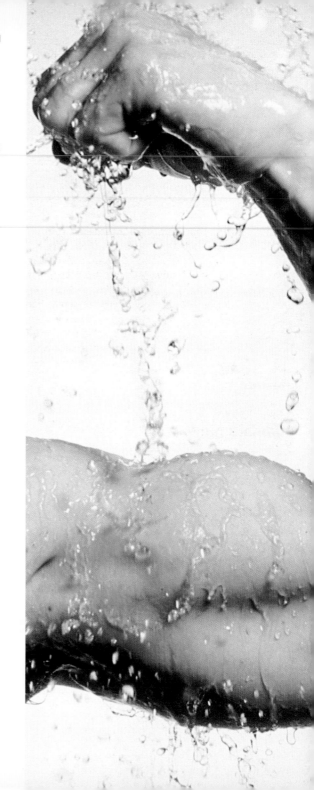

like gun metal. But don't overdo it: there is nothing less sexy than a man who spends hours in front of the mirror, especially when us women want to put our make-up on!

Not content with having their own moisturisers, men now want to rob women of their make-up. Maybe this has something to do with certain fashion designers, including Tom Ford of Gucci, sending 'made-up' men down the catwalk and getting rapturous applause for it. But unless you want to look like a drag queen, away from the catwalk the aim is to use make-up to enhance your features and camouflage any imperfections so that no one will have a clue that you are wearing any. All the conventional make-up rules apply to you, only more stringently. For example, ensure that you match your foundation and concealer to your skin tone; always blend well; and apply products such as loose powder to your hand before transferring them to your face.

When you're out shopping next, remember that it's not only make-up that you need to buy but also the tools – brushes, sponges and powder puffs. Items that you shouldn't be afraid to steal from women's make-up kits include: concealer, bronzing powder, eyebrow mousse, clear mascara, tinted moisturiser and foundation.

Unlike us girls, you guys don't need mountains of products to clutter up the bathroom or rob you of a month's salary. A couple of good basics – with the odd extra if your skin is playing up – and you're away. And you no longer need to beg, borrow or steal your favourite product, or face embarrassment by going to the women's cosmetics counter, as there are dozens of men's skincare preparations available, such as Philosophy's The Power Shower, Aveda's Shave Emollient, Aramis' Lab Series U-turn, Ralph Lauren's Shave Fitness Skin protecting Foam, MAC's NMF Moisture Regulating Emulsion, Clinique's M Shave Post Shave Healer, The Body Shop's Face Protector and Nivea's For Men Moisturising Lotion.

So what are the skincare essentials? A cleanser, in the form of a facial wash or cleansing bar (not soap) is a must to remove all the dirt and grime from your face. If, like most men, you wash your face in the shower, you may find multi-purpose hair, face and body washes more convenient. When it comes to shaving, a foam or gel is necessary if you wet-shave. Shaving should be followed by a moisturiser (also called skin balm) or a post-shave healer if your skin is particularly sensitive. Those prone to spots may want to consider using a cosmetics range specially designed for skin that tends to break out, as well as a spot-zapper for the odd zit. Added extras include a face scrub and lip balm but, in order to avoid losing your male identity altogether, use only the non-glossy balms. Finally, polish up your image by ensuring that nails are well-groomed and unwanted nose and ear hair is trimmed. And for the rest, flick through the pages of this book – you'd be surprised at how much applies to you.

SOS: QUICK FIXES FOR
THOSE BEAUTY EMERGENCIES

You want to look your very best but what happens? You wake up on that important morning only to discover a huge spot smack in the middle of your forehead, dark bags under your eyes and lips so sore that they look positively dry-roasted. There's no time for long-term solutions – you need a cure on the double!

SPOTS AND BLACKHEADS

Problem: a red, raw, pulsating pimple.

Solution: do not squeeze or touch the spot as this will aggravate it. Instead, dab on a healing spot lotion, such as Eve Lom's Dynamite lotion, Kiehl's Drying Paste, Desert Essence's Blemish Touch Stick or tea-tree essential oil. Take care to avoid overdrying it, or your pimple could become tricky to conceal. Before applying make-up, cover the spot with an antiseptic, non-greasy concealer, then set it with powder. Try The Body Shop's Tea-tree oil Cover Stick or Almay's Clear Balance Concealer. If your pimple is in a seductive place, why not take a brown eyeliner pencil and transform it into a beauty spot or stick one of Temptu's fake beauty spots over it? To remove unsightly blackheads, use a removal strip, such as Bioré's Pore Perfect Cleansing Strips, Ponds Clear Pore Strips or Elizabeth Arden's Pore-Fix C.

DRY PATCHES

Problem: patches of ultra-dry skin, caused by cold weather or central heating, that refuse to respond to your regular moisturiser.

Solution: firstly, remove any flaky skin by gentle exfoliation. Now apply a rehydrating mask to replace lost moisture and follow that with a rich moisturiser or urgent-moisture product. If your moisturiser is not rich enough, try using a blob of night cream. Alternatively, opt for one of the brilliant instant-remedy products on the market, such as Prescriptive's Flight Cream, Kiehl's Vit-E Ultra Moisturising Stick or Elizabeth Arden's Eight Hour Cream.

A SHINY FOREHEAD

Problem: a forehead that glistens and is so shiny that others can almost see their reflection in it; this could be the result of oily skin, hot weather or excess oil produced during your period.

Solution: apply one of the instant 'wonder' products which lap up oil, such as Philosophy's Never Let Them See You Shine, Decor's SOS Regulating Gel or Helena Rubinstein's Mat Specialist Shine Control. For a quick fix, blot with The Body Shop's Papier Poudre Oil Blotting Papers, Mister Mascara Japanese Rice Powder Block, Shiseido's Pureness Oil Blotting Paper or, for a DIY blotter, use kitchen paper.

SUNBURN

Problem: you've overdone the sunbathing and, as a result, look like a baked lobster.

Solution: cool and calm your skin down by resting a cold face cloth on the area for ten minutes. Remove cloth, and leave skin to breathe for a while before soothing and replenishing lost moisture with a lotion containing aloe vera or with a soothing product, such as Odely's

Soothing Gel Mask, Clarins' Aftersun Gel Ultra Soothing or Ambre Solaire's Instant Spray Relief. For a natural remedy, smear on the gel from the aloe vera plant. Diffuse redness by applying self-tanning lotion to the area or by using a green-tinted primer (also known as skin base or tint).

A DULL, TIRED COMPLEXION

Problem: a greyish-toned, dull-looking skin that lacks radiance.

Solution: restore your skin's natural glow with the following glow-boosters. Turn your head upside down to encourage blood flow; tap your face lightly with your index fingers for two minutes; splash your face with cold water; apply one of the following instant-radiance masks: Dior's Instant Radiance Relaxing Mask, Lancaster's Skin Therapy Oxygen Mask, Remède's Rescue Oxygen Mask or Revlon's Absolutes Energising Mask. Disguise a dull complexion with a light-reflecting foundation, then give your face a healthy glow with an instant colour-booster or bronzer, such as Kanebo's Exclusive Bio Bronzing Powder, Origins' Sunny Disposition, Nars' The Multiple or Guerlain's Divinaura.

BAD-HAIR DAYS

Problem: greasy, lank hair.

Solution: sprinkle a small amount of dry shampoo onto the roots, then brush it through. Appy a styling spray or volumising product and blast with the hairdryer.

Problem: hair that has fallen flat at the roots.

Solution: spritz styling spray or a volumising product onto the roots, turn your head upside down and blow-dry your hair. For extra lift, place a couple of large rollers at roots and leave for ten minutes. You could also gently backcomb your roots, then spritz with a holding spray. Another method is to pull up your hair into a ponytail and leave for ten minutes.

Problem: the moisture in the air has caused sleek hair to become frizzy, kinky or wavy.

Solution: dampen down your hair by spraying with a little water, then apply an anti-frizz serum and blow-dry.

TIRED EYES

Problem: dark circles, a puffy under-eye area and bloodshot eyes.

Solution: soothe your eyes and help alleviate redness by bathing them in an eye bath like Optrex's Eye Bath or Dr Hauschka's Eye Freshener Concentrate. Reduce dark circles and puffiness by placing chilled tea bags, cucumber slices or a purpose-made gel mask over your eyes and leave on for five minutes. Before you attempt to camouflage any dark circles, use Clarins' Skin Smoothing Eye Mask, Ultima II's Brighten Up, Tighten Up or Virgin Vie's Wide Awake Gel. Now cover the under-eye area with a good concealer, such as YSL's Touche Éclat, Bobbi Brown's Professional Concealer, BeneFit's Ooh La Lift or Clinique's Shadowliner. Keep eye make-up to a minimum: the trick is to draw attention away from your eyes, so go for soft colours and avoid harsh lines.

HIGH COLOUR OR BLUSHING

Problem: a bright-red face due to blushing that can make you wish the floor would swallow you up; a ruddy complexion; or high colour as a result of skin sensitivity.

Solution: cancel out redness by using a colour-corrective primer under your foundation. Good primers include Avon's Corrector Powder Pastels, Shiseido's Controlling Green Compact or Stick Foundation, MAC's Skin Tints or Shu Uemura's Base Control. If you don't wear foundation, try Decleor's Perfection du Teint which can be worn on its own.

CHAPPED LIPS

Problem: dry, crusty, chapped lips.

Solution: apply lashings of lip balm or Vaseline Petroleum Jelly to your lips, then exfoliate dead skin with a facial scrub, toothbrush, dry towel or lip-buffer, such as Colourings' Lip Scuff. Next, re-apply the balm. Must-have balms include Smith's Rosebud Balm, Kiehl's Lip Balm No 1, Eve Lom's Kiss Mix and WU!'s Ginseng and Royal Jelly Lip Balm.

BEAUTY THROUGH THE DECADES: FROM THE TEENS TO FIFTY-PLUS

This section guides you through the skincare, cosmetics, hairstyles and clothes for each decade of your life to help you to make the best of yourself, whatever your age.

THE TEENS

Plagued with inferiority complexes, hormonal changes, puppy fat and pimples, no wonder this decade is labelled 'the troublesome teens'. But the teenage years don't have to be so terrible: by eating well, staying active and keeping any skin break-outs under control you can enjoy this exciting period of your life. Do crazy things – you have years ahead of you when you'll have to conform. Experiment: plunder your mother's or big sister's make-up bag; play around with your hair and get acquainted with the make-up brush. Sit in front of a mirror with a magazine propped up next to you and try to copy a look that you like.

On a more serious note, as the majority of tooth decay occurs before you are twenty, you should make oral hygiene a priority. And if you haven't been blessed with even, straight teeth, now is the time to visit an orthodontist and get your teeth aligned. Because most sun damage is done before the age of eighteen, protecting yourself from the sun in your teens will also pay dividends later on in life. If you tower over your peers, the chances are that you will have a tendency to slouch. But it is important that you start standing straight as it is much easier to correct your posture now than after years of slouching. Back to age: you may yearn to be older, but remember that you are the envy of many women, so enjoy.

Cosmetics Don't overdo the make-up. The natural, 'barely-there' look is what you should aim to achieve, saving more glamorous looks for parties. Forget using any form of foundation

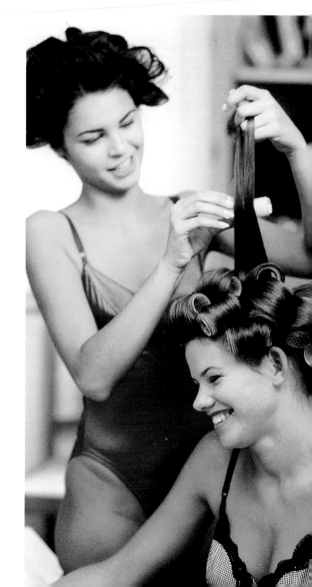

and instead stock up on neutral lip and eye colours for daywear, and inexpensive brightly-coloured eyeshadows, special-effect shimmer/glitter products and wacky lipsticks for partywear. On the skincare front, if you suffer from the typical teenager's greasy face and spots, keep these afflictions at bay by using an oil-control cleanser and anti-shine product, together with a gentle spot-zapper on the pimples.

Hair You may want to wear your tresses long and start experimenting with 'hair-up-dos' or, alternatively, break convention by sporting a head of pink spikes (though only if you are past school age, of course). Whatever you do, have fun with your hair.

Clothes Discover your own identity. This may mean flitting from one look to another or quickly developing one particular style, which could be anything from ethnic-style fashion to a military look. From a practical point of view, invest in a couple of good, supportive bras, not just the push-up types.

TWENTY-SOMETHING

Great! As you wave goodbye to the troublesome teens you find that you have blossomed into a beautiful young woman. No doubt you have stumbled across a hairstyle that suits you and, although you are still experimenting with make-up, you are more confident about applying it. Early twenties is when most women start their first serious job and, as a result, become more settled. Now is the time to schedule exercise into your routine, be it by joining a gym, taking part in a yoga class or prancing around in front of the TV to a supermodel's fitness video. To help maintain a svelte body, put your naughty student habits behind you and start eating the right foods. And, I'm afraid that those carefree times when you got away with staying up all night or falling into bed with your make-up on, are long gone.

Working hard and playing hard means that it's tempting just to slap a bit of moisturiser on, if and when you remember. But if you don't start looking after yourself, your neglect will catch up with you later on in life. Those who have until now only countenanced a trip to the beauty salon for waxing or an eyelash tint should consider regular facials to keep their skin clear and fresh-looking.

Cosmetics Your bathroom shelf will start to fill up as you add a few more products to your skincare basics. Invest in an eye gel and a light moisturiser to prevent premature ageing. Your skin is at its most resilient during your twenties, although your hormone levels can still be unsettled; if so use skincare preparations that will help to rebalance your complexion.

Hair Whether it's long, short or shoulder length, find a hairstyle that suits both your image and your lifestyle. Perhaps the time has come for you to pluck up the courage and have the long, girlish rats tails that you've cherished since you were ten cut into a more sophisticated style.

Clothes You're probably a slave to fashion magazines, but this is no bad thing: flicking through the fashion pages of *Vogue, Elle, Harper's Bazaar* and other glossies is a smart way in which to achieve a sense of style and an understanding of how to team outfits together. A word of wisdom: even if you are a self-confessed fashion victim, make sure that you choose clothes that flatter your shape.

THIRTY-SOMETHING

You've been dreading the big 3-0 for years, but once you've reached this milestone you'll quickly realise that it is, in fact, a wonderful time of your life. Elle Macpherson, Yasmin Le Bon, Brooke Shields, Linda Evangelista and Liz Hurley are all getting close to the thirty-five mark, yet they still have the faces and physiques of women a good decade younger.

In your thirties you have more self-confidence than ever before. You've got your act together, your emotions are more balanced and you know what suits you regarding hairstyles, make-up and clothes. But before you become too complacent, it is *vital* that you begin seriously investing in your looks or by the time you hit forty it will be too late.

As your sebaceous glands become less active, your skin's elasticity decreases, so your first line of defence should be stepping up your skincare routine: use a mask once a week and have a facial (or do your own home facial, see page 109) every four weeks. Get cracking with the facial exercises and stave off those sags, bags and dewlaps (see Eva Fraser's workout on page 106). With regard to body matters, bulges are far more difficult to budge when you are over thirty. And even if you are naturally slim, this is the time when breasts sag, cellulite takes hold and a podgy stomach sets in. Prevention is better than cure, so exercise regularly to keep your body well-toned, eat a healthy, well-balanced diet, and I promise that the investment will be worth it – especially when you pass for twenty-five! Finally, don't neglect your hands and neck; both show the tell-tale signs of age.

Cosmetics By all means start using serums and treatment masks, but rich, anti-ageing potions will be too heavy for you until you reach your mid- to late thirties. Skin texture can be improved by introducing a cosmecuetical to your skincare range, such as a Retin-A preparation (see page 100 for details). Stress can play havoc with your skin and you may find that you suffer from spots for the first time. Treat them with care, learn to relax and they will vanish almost as quickly as they appeared.

Hair You can wear your hair in almost any style, but if it's very long you may find that chopping off a few inches lops a few years off your age and gives you more sex appeal. If you are an over-bleached bottle blonde, soften any fake harshness by toning it down a shade, particularly if you wear your hair long.

Clothes By your thirties you should have developed your own individual style. If you've got a great figure there's nothing stopping you from wearing high-fashion numbers and still daring to show a bit of cleavage or glimpse of leg. But avoid that revealing-midriff-combined-with-a-minuscule-mini look: this type of outfit looks ridiculous on thirty-somethings. If you want to dress sexily and avoid looking tarty, go for figure-skimming numbers rather than something which looks like you've spent hours suffering to squeeze into it.

FORTY-SOMETHING

Life begins at forty – or so they say. And if Sharon Stone, Isabella Rossellini, Kim Basinger, Melanie Griffith and Michelle Pfeiffer are anything to go by, hitting forty doesn't mean that you have to look like a wizened old woman. In fact, if you take good care of yourself and have kind genes on your side there is no reason why you shouldn't look ten years younger.

At this stage in their lives, many women start rushing to the cosmetic surgeon. But rather than opt for the scalpel, you are still young enough to benefit from a range of less drastic age-reversal procedures on offer, such as laser treatments to zap wrinkles and retexturise the skin, and dermal fillers to plump out lines (see page 102). Make exercise a priority: it boosts the circulation, tones the skin, keeps you supple and will prevent sagging.

Cosmetics You are a cosmetics company's dream: there are more anti-ageing creams, serums and lotions to choose from than almost any other type of cosmetic on the market. As your skin becomes thinner and the production of sebum slows down, nourishing your skin is vitally important in order to forestall ageing. If your skin is very dry, use a wipe-off, oil-based cleanser. When it comes to make-up, less is most definitely more. Too much make-up highlights wrinkles and settles in lines, generally making you look years older.

Hair Covering grey hair is probably your prime concern. Grey hair can be elegant and flattering on a few women, but it tends to age most forty-somethings prematurely. As you grow older, your hair loses its volume, so start using thickening formulations or volumising mousses to improve its texture.

Clothes You've probably heard the expression 'mutton dressed as lamb' – avoid this label at all costs. Short skirts are permissible, but if you are still swanning around in your teenage ra-ra skirts, let's face it: you are stuck in a rut. Rather than trying to dress younger, enjoy injecting a touch of sophistication into your wardrobe. Build up a wardrobe of well-cut, good-quality clothes in superior fabrics.

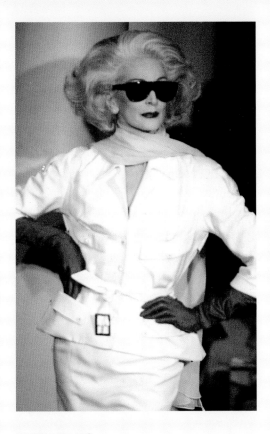

FIFTY-PLUS

Believe it or not, from fifty onwards you are probably less likely to be preoccupied with the race against time and more likely to feel comfortable with the way you look. By now you have no doubt gone grey, got wrinkles and have passed three of the dreaded decade marks. But don't fall into the trap of neglecting your appearance: it's never too late to be beautiful. Think of the gorgeous over fifties whom you can regard as role models, including Goldie Hawn, Lauren Hutton, Catherine Deneuve and mature model Carmen Dell'Orefice (see picture above). When it comes to your physique, unless you are seriously overweight avoid strict diets, and ensure that you are including 'good' fats (essential fatty acids) in your diet (see page 178). If you live off a diet of carrots and dry bread you will age considerably faster.

Take special care of your teeth: they are part of the skin's support. Once you lose them, your face will sink in and become hollow and wrinkled. Hormonal changes due to the menopause can cause your skin to become excessively dry or even oily, in which case you might find that you need to switch to a different range of skincare products. If you do decide to opt for surgery, you don't necessarily need a full face-lift, as there are many other procedures now available (see pages 102 and 138). Don't be tempted to bask in the sun thinking that the damage has already been done, otherwise your efforts to remain young looking will be futile.

Cosmetics The chances are that you are already hooked on the whole ensemble of anti-ageing creams, but as pigmentation can become irregular, you may want to use a whitening face cream to help even it out. And if you've noticed any of those little brown age spots creeping up on your skin, don't worry: you can fade them with the help of one of the better age-spot-zappers on the market. On the make-up front, switch to a rich, hydrating foundation but, to avoid accentuating wrinkles, keep it sheer.

Hair The question that bothers women over fifty is whether to continue colouring their hair or to let it go grey. This decision should depend on your particular shade of grey, which may be a flattering silver but, then again, could also be a lifeless dark grey. The general rule is, as you get older, it is more flattering to go lighter. Highlights add warmth, while a permanent tint will cover all traces of grey completely and is ideal if your hair is over sixty per cent grey.

Clothes Reassess your wardrobe. The sophisticated, dark colours or neutral tones that you wore in your thirties and forties might simply drain your face, so brighten up your appearance with a splash of colour. Forget flouncy dresses and pleated skirts, and wear streamlined shapes instead. Mid-calf-length skirts are decidedly ageing, so to avoid looking like granny, choose skirts that end just above the ankle or on the knee. If your specs are making you look older, update them. Finally, use your clothes to disguise floppy upper arms and scarves to conceal a 'turkey neck'.

STYLE

Take a vintage, tailored coat, a de-luxe cashmere top and a classic designer bag, add a pinch of creativity and lots of imagination – that's style. Read on and – you never know – you might make it on to the international best-dressed list!

Style is timeless – it never goes out of fashion and is not dictated by seasonal trends. Once you've found your personal style identity you don't have to torture yourself by trying to fit in with high fashion. This is not to say that style is immune to the dictate of fashion, or that the stylish are deeply unfashionable: a person who possesses style might be clad from head to toe in the season's hottest items or, alternatively, in classic pieces, vintage clothes, high-street numbers or a clever mixture of the lot.

Vogue fashion writer Mark Holgate believes that people with innate style possess that special 'X' ingredient: a discerning eye for clothes and an instinctive knowledge as to which items 'click'. 'The essence of style is about creative freedom, which means not being afraid to mix clothes from different sources and having the confidence to carry it off,' says Mark.

Like a painting or photograph, style is subjective, which makes it pretty difficult to quantify. In simple terms, it can be summed up as good dress sense. But don't be deceived into thinking that lavishing huge sums of money on designer gear will guarantee you a stylish appearance – someone could be stylish having spent a mere £1 in a thrift shop. So take some advice from *Allure* magazine's creative director, Polly Mellen, and don't think money. Putting cost aside for a moment, style is neither dependent on one item of clothing nor confined to any designer label. The stylish may mix Chanel with Gap, or high-street labels such as H&M with clothes found in a charity shop, for instance. It's how they team the pieces together to create the total look that matters. The same applies to interiors: it's not the individual chairs, curtains or colour of the walls that are stylish, it's the overall effect.

For those of you who exist in a permanent sartorial dilemma, it helps to remember that personal style doesn't happen overnight: it can, in fact, take years to cultivate. And don't forget that it's not just about getting the clothes right, but also about make-up, hair, jewellery, shoes and accessories. Mark points out that modern style has a great deal to do with juxtaposition. 'It's taking a dress and wearing it with the unexpected; it's playing items off against each other and striking contrasts. For example,

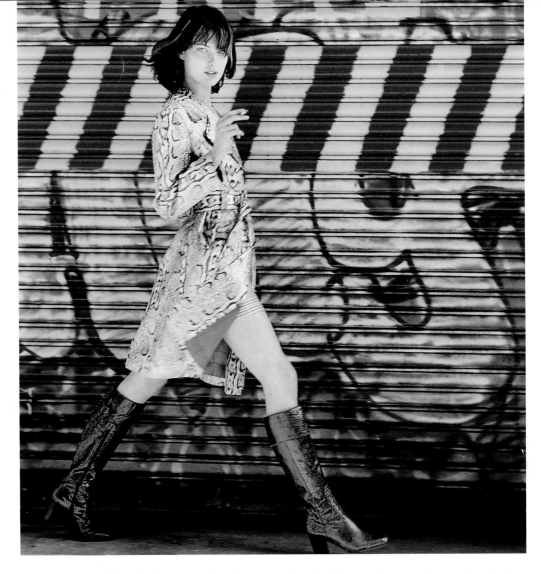

teaming an exquisite silk slip dress with a bare face as opposed to glossy make-up; scraping your hair back in an undisciplined way yet wearing dangly antique earrings; or teaming a denim jacket with a sequinned skirt.'

It may sound as though you can chuck on any old thing and – hey presto – style just happens (and we've all come across those sickeningly stylish folk who look resplendent in something they say they've just 'thrown on'). But what the stylish have in common is firstly, a love of clothes and, secondly, an understanding of the cut, shape, texture, length and fit of the garments and, of course, what works well together. Simplicity is the cornerstone of style: keep the look as simple as possible, for fussy is rarely stylish.

Finally, the ultimate style requisite is to look and feel totally at ease in whatever you wear, and to not look as though you've tried too hard. And be confident: or as *Allure*'s Polly Mellen so aptly puts it, 'Walk like a winner.'

STYLE IMPERATIVES

Not many people are lucky enough to have that Midas touch with clothes, so here are a few style pointers to help you let rip on your wardrobe and avoid any style *faux pas*. The ultimate aim is to create your own personal style – a strong look that transcends seasons, trends and occasions; an image that carries your stamp of identity without looking too stereotypical. To set your creative juices working, let me feed you a few key words from the style lexicon: freedom, simplicity, individuality and elegance. On the practical side, it's words like cut, colour, shape, quality, fit and finish that are synonymous with stylish dressing.

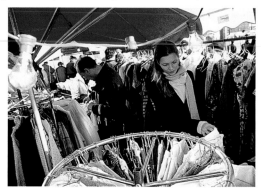
Kate Moss scours a Paris market for that special item.

- **Individuality**
Dressing with style means allowing your personality to shine through. If you give the same dress or shirt to two women, each would wear it in a different way, which is basically what individual style is all about. Take a little grey chiffon embroidered dress from a high-street store: one woman might wear it with chunky shoes and a jumper slung over the top, while the other with flamboyant heels and fancy jewellery. If you are clever with your hands, you can add an individual touch to your clothes by replacing buttons, adding a flower or beading, or turning an ugly dress into a great skirt.

- **Trademark elements** A smart trick that you can learn from models, celebrities and style aficionados is to wear one special item so frequently that it becomes your signature piece. Whether it's a shawl, an ornate bag, a white shirt, a wacky hat or antique earrings, make this item the main ingredient of your personal style.

Inspiration To prevent yourself buying another fashion blunder, gather inspiration before you even step your Manolo heel on the shop floor. You'll find it in all kinds of places – while watching old movies, diving into past fashions through the catalysts of history books and museums, and scouring the fashion pages of such magazines as *Vogue*, *Elle* and *Marie Claire*. The catwalk is also inspirational, but don't take it too literally or you'll be walking down the street in what looks like a perspex shower curtain.

- **Sources** The stylish sift through second-hand designer stores, thrift shops, markets, high-street chains, classic-knitwear shops and jumble sales. They also check out their grandmother's dressing-up box and readily accept hand-me-downs from their parents or grandparents. While on their travels, they keep an eye open for kaftans, sarongs, ethnic jewellery and other native pieces. So wherever you are in the world, be it the Himalayas or the Highlands, look out for clothes: who knows, you might come back from your trip to a remote fishing village with a divine, hand-knitted jumper!

- **Mix** Whether you favour the minimalist end of the fashion spectrum to a more eclectic style, or like to cross-fertilise the two, the key to looking *à la mode* is clever mixing and juxtaposition: take a cardigan and skirt, for example, these garments may work together or could make you look like you dressed while blindfolded. Aside from the mixing of the actual style of the garments, you may want to stick to the latest fashions or mix part modern with part classic or part vintage.

TOP STYLE TIPS

- **Dress with timeless style**. Effortless classics are more fool-proof than high fashion, so invest in a few indispensable staples, such as a crisp, white shirt, T-shirts, a simple, fitted cardigan, easy shift dresses and streamlined trousers.

- The trick to **updating your look** is to inject your wardrobe with a few contemporary pieces. You don't have to go the whole hog: simply introduce the latest colour or the hottest pair of shoes to your wardrobe.

- As fashion is cyclical and keeps regurgitating and reworking past trends, you'd be wise to **hold onto any great pieces**. This way you can look to your own fashion archives for inspiration.

- **Intelligent dressing** means dressing appropriately – taking your lifestyle and its constraints into consideration, and striking a balance between fashion and wearability.

- Use your clothes to **accentuate your good points** and de-emphasise the bad. Decide which styles flatter your shape and stick to them, ignoring trends if they don't suit you.

- What looks fabulous on the hanger could make you look like a bag lady. **Always try on clothes before you buy** them, and remember that they should fit like a glove and hang well.

- Accessories should always be pared down to avoid overkill: **stick to one fabulous, classic piece**.

- **Vary the textures of your garments** with interesting fabrics, like bouclé, linen, crochet, velour, cashmere, felt, fake fur and PVC. And add a touch of opulence to your wardrobe with such exquisite fabrics as silk, velvet and lurex.

- When out shopping, don't become dispirited. **Sizes vary enormously**: what is a large size 10 in one shop might be a small size 14 in another.

- **Inject colour into your wardrobe**. Use bright hues to punctuate your look, but avoid wearing hard-to-wear shades too close to your face or you could end up looking positively sick. When wearing varying shades of the same colour, make sure that they complement each other – unless clashing is intentional!

- **Black is stylish and slimming** and has been the uniform of fashion editors, stylists and models for years, but overdo it and it becomes a lazy, uninspiring option. To avoid looking like you are going to a funeral, accent black with colour, white or neutral tones. When shopping for black garments, pay attention to the cut and fabric.

- Always take **the comfort factor** into consideration when buying clothes: if a skirt is so tight or shoes are so high that you can hardly walk, you will 'cramp' every ounce of your style.

- The best way of finding out **what's in** is to look through the fashion magazines. But rather than slavishly copy an outfit piece by piece, the trick is to adapt the look to what suits you.

- The high-street chains are indispensable when it comes to finding **cheap, stylish numbers**. The quality is, however, reflected in the price, so check for wonky hems and necklines, darts in the wrong places and bulky seams.

- For **maximum fashion mileage**, it's worth spending a little extra on tailored items, such as jackets, coats and trousers, as both the cut and quality of the fabric will be superior.

STYLISH DRESSERS

Who are the 'style-sussed', what do they wear, where do they shop and what makes them so decidedly stylish? Here are the answers.

STYLISH LOOKS

For the purpose of creating some sort of definition and distinction – and at the risk of losing any fashion kudos that I might possess and having to hang up my Guccis for good – I shall dare loosely to categorise the stylish into two groups. (But remember that each group has dozens of variations.)

The first group consists of the impeccably-dressed brigade, which favours pared-down, modern classics – 'simplicity' is the word that gets them writhing around in excitement. These minimalists dress in a polished yet understated way, sporting clean lines and good-quality fabrics. Put simply, they wear elegant, unadorned clothes that are wearable enough for the office. Their mantra of 'no fuss, no nonsense' results in a relaxed yet co-ordinated look that is slick, smart and incredibly chic.

Group two comprises those hip dressers who have a more eclectic edge. This look screams unconventionality: funky one minute, feminine in floaty chiffon with chunky heels the next. It's all about mix and mismatch. Devotees of vintage chic, hip dressers carefully 'throw' their clothes together to look creative, arty, cultured, well travelled and therefore utterly cool.

Where the stylish shop Lingerie shops (for underwear as outerwear), second-hand designer stores, antique markets, charity shops, designer diffusion boutiques, kids' shops (for T-shirts and little cardigans), high-street chains (for high-fashion numbers), shopping villages (for cut-price designer clothes), army-surplus stores and department stores (for basics).

The stylish To help you picture someone with style, here are a few renowned stylish dressers (past and present). Audrey Hepburn, Diana Vreeland, Jemima Khan, Juliette Binoche, Courtney Love, Cate Blanchette, Julia Roberts, Anna Wintour, Shalom Harlow, Lauren Bacall, Liv Tyler, Cameron Diaz, Minnie Driver, Madonna, Jennifer Lopaz, Yasmin Le Bon, Winona Ryder, Natalie Imbruglia, Uma Thurman, Jo Levin, Kate Moss, Erin O'Connor, Karen Elson, Jackie Onassis, Nicole Kidman, Naomi Campbell, Gwyneth Paltrow, Polly Mellen, Aerin Lauder, Julia Ormand, Calista Flockhart, Sophie Dahl, Mica Paris, Amanda de Cadenet, Jade Jagger, Isabella Blow, Princess Caroline of Monaco, Patsy Kensit, Donatella Versace, Catherine Deneuve, Jenny McCarthy, Grace Kelly, Jennifer Aniston, Carolyn Bessette Kennedy, Denise van Outen, Grace Coddington, Susie Bick, Stella Tennant, Kristin Scott Thomas and Helena Christensen.

What the stylish wear Helmet Lang, Voyage, H&M, Alexander McQueen, John Galliano, Vivienne Westwood, French Connection, Manolo Blahnik, Kookai, Tocca, Emma Hope, Gucci, Prada, Mui Mui, Clements Ribero, Antonio Beradi, Marc Jacobs, Stella McCartney, Matthew Williamson, Yohji Yammamoto, Anna Sui, Oasis, Leiney Keogh, Hermes (for bags), Betsey Johnson, Agent Provocateur, Gap, Levi's, Isaac Mizrahi, Narcisco Rodringuez, Calvin Klein and Ann Demeulemeester.

Opposite page: Supermodel Helena Christensen, who has been voted one of the most sylish women, is a great example of model style.

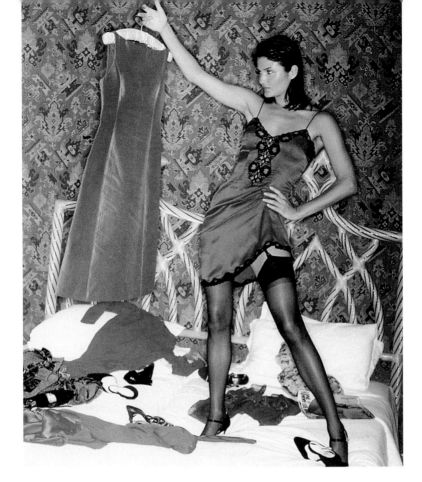

MODEL STYLE

Let's take a look at those arbiters of good taste – models. But don't be fooled: you won't see 'model style' on the catwalks or in the magazines – it's what you see off set that counts. When a model slopes into the studio or is chilling out backstage at the shows, this is when you'll see the true reflection of 'model style'. 'I think the fact that models have become style icons has a lot to do with them being photographed backstage in their own clothes,' says *Vogue* fashion writer Mark Holgate. 'And, as they are dressed up and styled everyday, it makes sense for them to be passionate about clothes. In fact, models have such a strong and individual style that designers are turning to *them* for inspiration these days.'

Models have always been at the forefront of style. Until recently they tended to encapsulate the most dominant look of each era, like Twiggy in the 1960s, or the supermodels in the early nineties, when almost any model worth her day rate would be dressed from head-to-toe in Chanel, Versace, Alaïa or another A-list designer. But despite being surrounded by designer clothes, these days you'll rarely see a model dressed from head to toe in one label unless it's for a glitzy bash, and then it's more likely be an original Halston or vintage Yves Saint Laurent. Whether it's an evening frock or simple cardi, their aim is to wear something that no one can identify. Call it intuitive, but models appear to know that too much of one label, or overdosing on designer gear, can dissipate personal style.

STYLE QUEENS

To assist me with the near-impossible task of picking three of the world's most stylish women, I enlisted the help of *Vogue* fashion writer Mark Holgate.

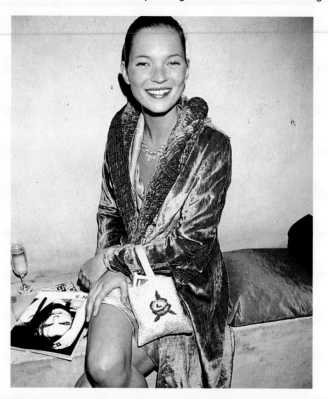

SUPERMODEL WITH STYLE

This British supermodel, who first personified grunge in the early 1990s, went on to become arguably *the* style icon of the 1990s. According to Mark, Kate Moss rarely throws anything out: like a magpie, she collects fabulous pieces from different sources, storing and later reworking them. Her favourite haunts are thrift shops and second-hand designer stores, and she has a penchant for beautiful jewellery. 'Kate always looks finely honed,' enthuses Mark. 'She loves clothes and understands them. Her trademark is clever juxtaposition. She'll scrape her hair back and go bare-faced while wearing an ultra-feminine Galliano dress, or she might jazz up denim with kitten heels and diamonds. Kate oozes that British quirkiness. You'll see her in some stunning outfit, but you are never quite sure who it's by or where she got it from.'

FASHION PRO WITH STYLE

A devotee of Ralph Lauren by day and of Chanel by night, *GQ* magazine's fashion director, Jo Levin, is a minimalist dresser who has one strong look, yet every now and again wows everyone around her by wearing something devilishly unpredictable. Working in fashion means that it's tempting to change your look constantly. But Jo isn't a slave to seasonal fads: in fact, she has a penchant for 1950s-style clothes which, she says, suit her figure. Like most style queens, Jo has a signature piece that she is rarely seen without: her pearl necklace. According to Mark, she is very comfortable with her own style: 'Jo shows up to work wearing simple, pared-down trousers with a crisp, white shirt or classic cashmere jersey. Then, out of the blue, she will turn up in something totally unexpected. It is this element of surprise, and not being afraid to change, that makes Jo impossibly stylish.'

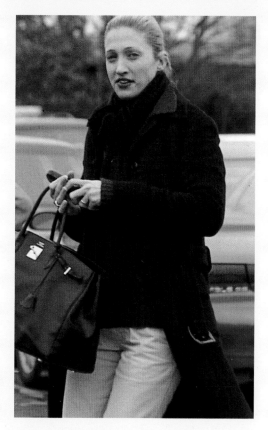

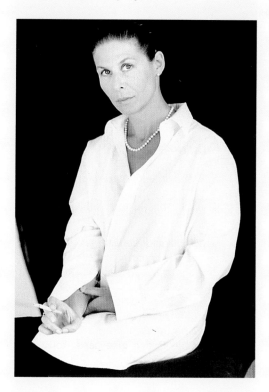

CELEBRITY WITH STYLE

Labelled 'the style queen of America', Carolyn's customary chic led to a demand for her to launch her own range of clothes – CBK. Her trademark is simplicity: clean lines, neutral colours and definitely no fuss. Wearing smart casuals, she always looks elegant, no matter where she goes. 'This woman clearly knows how to dress,' comments Mark. 'Whether she's wearing Calvin Klein, Prada or Narcisco Rodringuez, her style is clean and pared down. And she is one of those rare creatures who wears jeans with heaps of style. She'll team them with strappy evening shoes and a simple sweater – yet she'll look great. But the most important thing about Carolyn is that, no matter what she wears, she never lets the clothes overshadow her.'

KISS AND MAKE UP

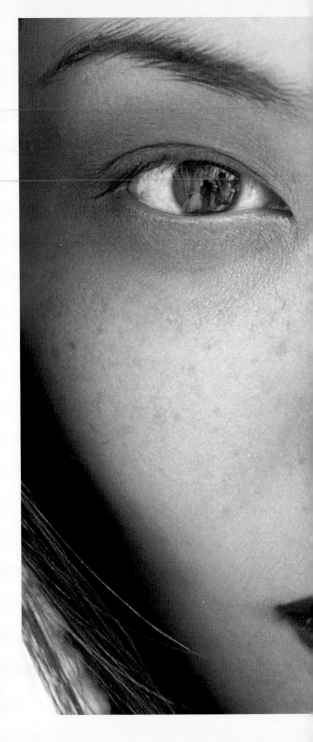

Whether you are painted to the hilt, or are the type who's never quite got to grips with what's right for you, these make-up superhints will help you to get well acquainted with the lipstick, powder and paint.

Even if it's just a smidgen of concealer or a swift slick of lip gloss, make-up gives you a polished look and enhances your features. It can make lips fuller, eyes bigger and skin flawless – it's also handy for camouflaging imperfections. And, if you are in need of a total transformation, make-up can play a part in that, too.

No longer solely confined to the beauty counter, make-up is both user-friendly and widely available: you can pop into your local supermarket for a loaf of bread and come out with a scarlet lipstick or, while scouring shops for clothes, drop into a make-up emporium such as MAC, ScreenFace and Sephora and pick up an iridescent eyeshadow. But the primary factor that should put make-up high on your beauty agenda is that, according to top make-up artist Vincent Longo, today's cosmetics are easier to apply than ever before: 'Clever applicators, swivel-ups, push-up pencils, make-up sticks and brand-new textures that glide easily on to the skin mean that women can make up with convenience and ease.' Many people are under the illusion that the more expensive the item of make-up the better the results. You don't need to break the bank, however, especially on items that are not part of your everyday make-up kit. It's more a case of if it works for you – buy it.

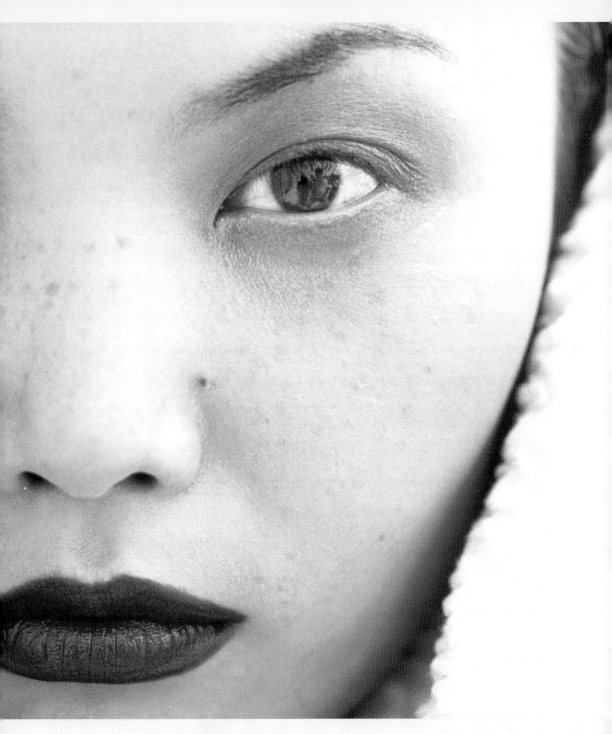

THE MAKE-UP PALETTE

TIPS ON THE RIGHT SHADES

Leading make-up artist Trish McEvoy, who has her own signature range, helps you choose the best shades of make-up for your colouring.

Redheads: 'Stick with a foundation that has more warmth in it to cancel out some of your natural ruddiness. The blush tones that work best are in the peachy-bronze colour group. For your eyes, use vanilla-cream-coloured eyeshadow accented with terracotta, and a dark brown to line your eyes. Mascara should be dark brown or black. Colour your lips in shades of browns and soft corals (like our #1).'

Blondes: 'Foundation that incorporates your skin's natural undertones into it is best. Choose a blush colour that mimics the naturally flushed colour you get from a brisk walk in the park. Brown or black mascara works best, along with soft and neutral-toned eye colours, preferably soft bieges, taupes and browns. For lips, use satiny brown-pinks or soft-brown tones with a nude lip liner (like our #12).'

Brunettes: 'Find a foundation that can correct some sallowness that might be present in your skin tone; use a warm or neutral shade. The blushes that work best are a mixed palette of bronze and dusty pinks with a touch of coral. Emphasise your eyes with black mascara, and choose eyeshadow in redwood-chestnut and bronze shades to bring out the natural highlights and tones that already exist in your hair colouring. Lip colour from the red/brown family (like our Lip Essential Kit #11) is most flattering.'

TIPS ON CHOOSING MAKE-UP

Top make-up artist Jeanine Lobell, who is the woman behind the cult make-up range Stila, believes that one of the best ways in which to find a look that suits you is to visit a professional make-up artist: 'Go to your nearest specialist store and book a consultation. Choose a brand that employs trained artists rather than just sales people. Look for make-up artists that present themselves in a way that looks good to you. Don't just try one consultation – try two or three and see if there are common elements in the looks that work well for you, discarding any that you don't like. Ask to try different make-up and find out why the artists use certain products and not others. When you've found a product you like, always check the colour in good light – daylight, if possible, to see the real shade.'

YOUR MAKE-UP WARDROBE

Vincent Longo, a make-up supremo who has his own range, believes that every woman should have a make-up kit/wardrobe containing a selection of different choices for day-, evening-, and partywear. It's not about finding one eyeshadow or one lipstick that you like and rigidly sticking to it: vary your make-up to suit your clothes, the season, your mood, the location and the occasion. 'You wouldn't have only one dress for evening and one pair of trousers for day, now would you?' muses Vincent. 'Create your basic make-up blueprint, then add to it. Have the season's hottest and trendiest items by all means, but invest in different textures and colours so that you can switch.' Review your make-up wardrobe every few months by cleaning out your make-up bag and throwing away any old, gungy make-up.

PREPARE TO MAKE UP

The secret of beautiful make-up lies in the application – it's your features that you want to leap out from your face not your make-up, so practice until you get it right. Each morning before you pick up your make-up brush, look at the face that is staring at you from the mirror and decide what you need to apply, rather than slapping on the same lipstick, powder and blush day in, day out. Perhaps you have benefited from a good night's sleep and therefore require little, if any, foundation. On the other hand, having drunk one too many G & Ts and had a late night you may be looking pasty and need the full works!

A fool-proof application requires a steady hand, so rest your elbow on a table. Be it eyeshadow, blush or foundation, the golden rule is to blend, blend, blend. Whenever possible, apply your make-up in natural daylight and check it under different lights before you leave the house.

DAY-TO-EVENING TRANSFORMATION

You can simply fast-forward to evening by defining your features with brighter, bolder or more sumptuous colours, or by wearing iridescent textures. When it comes to foundation, as evening light is generally softer and more flattering than daylight, opt for a sheer rather than a heavy-weight texture. Tuck a highlighter stick into your make-up bag and sweep it across your brow bones or cheekbones, and add a slick of gloss to your lips for a touch of glamour.

THE NATURAL LOOK

Also known as 'barely-there', 'naked enhancement' or 'nude', the object of a natural look is to give the impression that you are a fresh-faced, untampered-with beauty. Soft neutral colours, such as beige or tawny shades for your eyes, rosy for cheeks and flesh-coloured or terracotta tones for your lips, work well. Pencils and powders are best for eyes as they create a softer effect. For adding a hint of colour without coverage, stains are ideal because they impart a natural rosy glow to the cheeks, lips and brow bones. If you want to cover blemishes, do so with either concealer, a light covering of tinted moisturiser or a sheer foundation, so as not to mask the skin's natural shine.

BETTER BASES

Foundation and tinted-moisturiser tips The purpose of applying a base is to smooth out any flaws and make your skin appear even-toned. Base is not meant to cover your face like a mask, yet the biggest mistake that most women make is to cake it on, which looks unnatural and ends up accentuating rather than disguising any skin flaws. • When buying a base, don't scrimp: invest in a good-quality product that matches your skin tone exactly. Test the product on your face, not your hand, and check the result in daylight before purchasing it. • Some make-up artists apply base with their fingers, while others use a sponge; whichever method you prefer, ensure that you blend well and smooth out any tell-tale lines around your jaw and hairline. • If you have dry skin, you should use a hydrating oil-based foundation, while if you have an oily, combination or spotty skin, you should opt for an oil-free mattifying foundation which will keep oil at bay and is less likely to clogg the pores. • You don't need to apply base all over your face, only to the parts that need it. • For a more natural look, use tinted mosturiser rather than foundation. • Two-in-one foundation/powder compacts give a lighter coverage than liquid foundation and are great for touch-ups.

Powder tips Powder sets foundation and concealer, and comes in two forms: pressed and loose. Loose powder gives better coverage, while pressed powder is ideal to carry in your handbag for touch-ups. • When applying loose powder, dip a velour powder puff, paddle brush or big, fluffy make-up brush into the pot before transferring the powder to the back of your hand. Tap the brush or give the puff a final shake before brushing or pressing the powder onto your face. • In order to avoid that obvious powdery, matt look, a little is all that's needed. • Brush downwards to prevent the powder clogging up on your facial hairs. • Bronzing powders will give you that sun-kissed look, but go sparingly, as they can look too obvious.

CLEVER CONCEALING

Concealing tips Concealer can be used to cover blemishes, dark under-eye circles, the area along the side of each nostril and as a primer for eyeshadow. • Choose a concealer that is one or two shades lighter than your skin tone (but don't use too light a one under your eyes or you'll end up with obvious circles). • Foundation can also be used as a concealer – opt for one that is a shade lighter than your normal foundation or your skin tone. • To prevent concealer collecting in the creases under your eyes, apply eye cream first. • Always set your concealer with a light dusting of powder. • When covering spots, the aim is to make the spot's colour appear as close to your skin tone as possible.

BLUSHING BEAUTY

Blush tips Apply powder blush with a large, fluffy brush; transfer from the pot to the back of your hand first, remove any excess blush off the brush, then sweep it on in movements towards your ear. • If you've been rather heavy-handed, defuse the blush with some loose, translucent powder. • For razor-sharp-looking cheekbones, sweep a little bronzing or contour powder underneath your cheekbones before highlighting the cheekbones themselves with a touch of shimmer or iridescent ivory eyeshadow.

• To brighten your eyes, dust blush across your brow bones. • When applying cream or gel blushes, blend with your fingers, using circular movements. • For a rosy glow, apply blush only to the apples of your cheeks (ignoring your cheekbones). • Powder blush sits better on a base, whereas cream and gel blushes work on both naked skin and base. • Stains give a healthy wash of colour and are long-lasting.

ALL EYES

Eyeshadow tips Whether you want Mohican-style bands or a dainty line, be aware that even the tiniest amount of make-up will enhance your eyes. • Before you start colouring your eyes, always prime your upper-eye area (including your lids) with foundation or concealer; your make-up will stay put longer. • Unless you want a colourful effect, use eyeshadow in soft, flattering, neutral shades. • In order to prevent bits of it landing on your face, when applying eye make-up hold a piece of tissue under your eyes and always shake off any excess powder from the brush before applying it. • To open up your eyes, sweep pale eyeshadow (such as ivory) over your brow bone.

Eyeliner tips Define your eyes using one of the various shades of brown, or charcoal-grey, navy or black eyeliner. • A kohl pencil is easy to use and the effect can be softened with a brush or cotton bud. • Eyeshadow used as a liner gives a softer, more natural, look. You can also use eyeshadow to soften any obvious lines. • Liquid liner looks harsh and requires a steady hand and lots of practice, so keep a cotton bud handy to correct any mistakes. Liner pens are more fool-proof. • Unless you want racoon-like eyes, don't apply liners or eyeshadows too low under your eyes. • To elongate your eyes, take the eyeliner from the centre of your pupil to the outer corners of your upper eyelids.

Lash tips If you want to apply more than one coat of mascara, allow the first to dry before applying the next. • To make your lashes appear thicker, dust them with powder before applying mascara. • Black, dark-brown and brown mascaras work best; you should limit coloured mascaras for parties, or just brush them onto the tips of your lashes. • For mascara that lasts, use either a long-lasting or a water-resistant mascara. • Clear mascara is ideal for a natural look and also holds curled lashes in place.

BEAUTIFY YOUR BROWS

Eyebrow tips From dominant, Brook Shields-like eyebrows to Kate Moss' sparse slivers, groomed eyebrows can make a big difference to your face and can also open up your eyes. • Define your brows with an eyebrow-definer, eyebrow pencil or eyeshadow, using feather-light strokes. • If you are very fair, fill in your brows with a taupe- or beige-coloured pencil. • Keep your eyebrows in place with brow mousse, clear mascara or a slick of Vaseline Petroleum Jelly.

SLICK LIPS

Lip tips Lip colour no longer simply means a lipstick: it could also be a gloss, stain or pencil. To confuse you further, there is now a plethora of finishes, including satin, matt, frosted, glossy, opalescent and sheer. Colour-wise, you can choose from a kaleidoscope of shades from ravishing reds to demure browns, or simply opt for a flesh-coloured shade. • Before applying lip colour, always prime your lips with lip balm. • Create your own custom-made lip colour by blending a couple of shades together. • To make your lips appear bigger, outline them with a concealer or foundation-coated lip brush, and then a flesh-coloured, matt lip pencil before applying lipstick; if you want to enlarge your lips by taking the line outside your natural lip line, do so only fractionally or the result will be too obvious. • To give the illusion of a pouting mouth, dab a tiny dot of lip gloss to the centre of your bottom lip. • For precision, apply lipstick with a brush. • If you prefer to wear gloss instead of lipstick, use a flesh-coloured lip pencil

on the entire lip, then apply the gloss with a brush. Colouring the lip in pencil also makes a good base for lipstick. • For longer-lasting lip colour, apply one layer of colour, then blot your lips and reapply. Alternatively, choose a long-wear lipstick or coat with a lip fix.

TRICKS TO MAKE YOU LOOK YEARS YOUNGER

If not applied correctly, or too heavily, make-up can age you. • Go carefully with concealer: it has a habit of settling in lines and making them look more prominent. • Less is always more when it comes to base. • When choosing a foundation, look for a sheer, light-reflective formulation that softens the appearance of wrinkles. • As you get older, your skin tone changes, so check that your foundation is still a good match. • Powder can accentuate wrinkles, therefore a light dusting is all that's needed. • Refrain from wearing draining eyeshadow colours – choose soft neutrals (warm beiges, taupes and browns) instead. • Go easy on the mascara and don't coat your bottom lashes – there's nothing more ageing than the spidery, clogged-lash effect. • Lipstick tends to seep into those nasty, vertical lines above the top lip, so prime your lips before applying it. Use a lip barrier, such as BeneFit's Degroovy, which will help prevent bleeding, or lock in your lip colour by outlining your lips with a flesh-coloured lip pencil first. Avoid obvious lines, as lips outlined in a colour darker than your lipstick not only looks dated, it's also ageing. • Use brushes to apply your make-up and blend like mad, softening any hard lines with a cotton bud. • A few of the age-defying ranges and products on the market include Ultima II's Line Smoothing Foundation, Dior's Teint Actuel Line Softening Make-up, Laura Mercier's Moisturizing Foundation and Revlon's Age Defying Make-up.

RUNWAY-STYLE MAKE-UP

It's fantastic, it's frivolous and it's fun. Here are some backstage tips which will help you to upstage others with your show-stopping make-up.

Make-up maestro François Nars believes that runway-style make-up is a great way in which to freshen up your look. 'Not everyone can rush out and buy the latest Versace outfit, but by trying some of the season's new make-up techniques you can add new life to your current look', says Nars, who has applied his signature palette to the face of almost every supermodel and dozens of celebrities, including Julia Roberts and Sharon Stone. 'Runway looks are an inspiration. The best show make-up will suggest new ways that you can play with your own look and encourage you to experiment with your usual style.'

Warpaint-style stripes, black lips and gold faces – catwalk make-up is decidedly cutting edge. And much of the time it's pure fantasy or, as Nars puts it, 'fashion masturbation': 'Designers, make-up artists and hair stylists are not thinking about what real women want, they are just pleasing themselves,' he muses, continuing: 'Catwalk make-up is usually extreme. Although not necessarily strong and dramatic (sometimes it can be an almost completely bare face), it is designed to create an effect. The worst thing about trying to copy runway make-up is that it is so easy to make mistakes. Not all runway work is really beautiful in any case – even on the most amazing model, so even the most brilliant version of such a look is not going to look good for normal wear.'

It's the faces painted for the catwalk that provide the direction for each season's new make-up trends. So what of the future? Will we be seeing one strong trend or a variety of themes transcending from the runways? According to Nars, there is no longer one single make-up look that dominates: 'Freedom is the only dictate into the new millennium.'

GET THE LOOK

With the ever-growing number of make-up artists' signature ranges, like Nars, Vincent Longo, Bobbi Brown, Stila and Trish McEvoy, all the tools of the catwalk are now available for you to use at home. And, with these key elements from the runways, you can give your make-up that supermodel edge.

Be inspired

'Women should see what is happening on the runways and be inspired', points out Nars. 'But I don't want them to copy exactly what they see. Instead, they should tailor it to their own individual style.' Take your cue from Nars: be influenced and inspired by the make-up you see in catwalk shots and footage, but don't attempt to reproduce a hard-to-wear effect that could look simply hideous on you.

Take a single element

You can add a modern edge to your make-up by taking inspiration from a single component of a runway trend, such as a colour, texture or technique. For example, pick a lip colour, reinterpret a eyeshadow application or invest in a new textured base. By simply varying the strength of application, make-up artists achieve different looks: a hint of blush to create a rosy glow will give a completely different look to the bright, exaggerated sweeps of colour that sit on the cheekbones. Whatever element you choose, adapt it to suit your features or you could end up looking like you have been rather heavy handed or, what's worse, incredibly dated. Retro looks are often seen on the runways, but they still have a contemporary twist that brings them up to date.

Become colourful

Brightly coloured make-up has appeared on the runways for several seasons and looks like it's here to stay. Eye make-up has the most mileage when it comes to colour, so reserve paint-box-bright hues, such as yellow, turquoise, lilac, green and pastel blue, for your eyes. While neutrals are a piece of cake to apply, colour is not quite such a doddle. In order to avoid looking like a cabaret artist, go carefully on the application, applying a little at a time and blending well. If you're going for washes of colour on your eyes or are using coloured mascara, keep your lips neutral. (You may want to stick to brown or black mascara and just sweep a touch of coloured mascara to the tips of your lashes.) Only allow one feature to take centre stage. If you prefer to brighten up your pout with such tantalising hues as burnt orange and berry red, accent your eyes in muted shades.

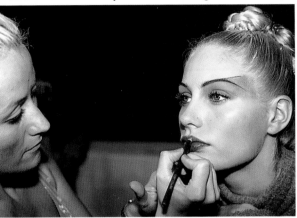

smudge a touch of gold over your eyelids or slick it over your lipstick as a final touch; add glitter to your eye make-up or along your brow bones.

Shimmer

The fashion world witnessed an incandescent moment when every model on every catwalk glistened from head to toe, not with droplets of sweat, but with particles of shimmer products worn on different areas of the face and body. Iridescent make-up remains a mainstay element, albeit in a more subtle, pared-down way. It can be used in a multitude of ways from highlighting cheekbones and opening up eyes to creating an all-over glow. However, shimmery bases and blush have a habit of highlighting the good, the bad and the ugly, so give them a miss if you have any spots or blemishes. The body products are more forgiving and are great for evening, so let your shoulders, arms, legs or décolletage glisten.

False eyelashes

False eyelashes are catwalk favourites, and also work well for clubbing and partying. Paint them with coloured mascara or, for an even wider choice of colour, with nail polish.

Special effects

The catwalk is a brilliant source of inspiration for a variety of special effects: glitter, metallic face paints and beauty spots made from jewels, stars or hearts, for example. You'll find little pots of such fancy stuff in make-up and fashion boutiques or department stores. But while special effects are perfect for clubs and parties, don't overdo it (unless, that is, you want to look like you've just taken part in a Christmas pantomime). Again, it's about taking one element and reinterpreting it to work with the rest of your make-up. For example:

Update your make-up

One problem that many women encounter is getting stuck in a make-up time-warp. But you wouldn't still wear those psychedelic hot pants that you wore in your teens, would you? So if you are guilty of slapping on the same old lipstick, mascara or foundation, it's definitely time for a make-up overhaul. Besides, updating your make-up kit is essential, not just for fashion's sake, but also to take advantage of the latest textures which sit more comfortably on the skin and last longer. Scour the fashion and beauty stories in magazines for the season's catwalk must-haves. After that, your first stop should be the cosmetic counter or make-up boutique. You don't need to buy a completely new set of make-up – one or two hot items is all it takes to update your make-up wardrobe and achieve a runway look.

FRANÇOIS NARS' TOP-TEN TIPS FOR RUNWAY-INSPIRED EVENING MAKE-UP

1 Never apply too much make-up: more is not better for evening. Modern make-up is sheer, even for evening, so layering on more make-up will just make the look appear dated.

2 Add a bit of shimmer to your brow bones, the tops of your cheeks and the centre of your lips. (Nars' The Multiple, in either Copacabana or South Beach, provides a perfectly sheer shimmer with which to accent your skin tone softly.)

3 Add lip gloss: apply a clear shade over your favourite lipstick for glamour or use a coloured lip gloss for a moist, sexy mouth. Because it catches the light, gloss helps to make the lips appear fuller. (Try Nars' Triple X.)

4 Always perfect the outline of your lips with a lip-liner pencil. In addition to enhancing the shape of your lips, lining them helps lipstick to stay on longer, particularly throughout dinner.

5 Pick one feature – your eyes or lips, perhaps – and play it up. Smoky eyes should be teamed with a soft, more natural-looking mouth. Conversely, when wearing a deep lipstick, keep your eye make-up to a minimum. Apply a beige or white, transparently pearled shade to add sparkle and light to your eyes, then smudge a bit of pencil close to the base of your lashes to provide definition. That should be all that you will need with dark lips, for too much eye make-up will overdo the look.

6 Waterproof mascara will stay in place for longer and will not flake or smudge.

7 Avoid using a dark foundation: choosing a lighter shade, which matches your skin or is one shade lighter, will help your skin to glow.

8 Choose a concealer that is a bit lighter than your skin tone for your eye area. Eliminating any dark circles and illuminating this area will help your eyes to look brighter.

9 Go gently on the blush. Using a soft, translucent blush liberally, rather than overloading your cheeks with a dark shade, will create warmth.

10 Use an eyelash curler to perk up your eyes.

The products mentioned are from Nars' own signature make-up line which, contained as it is in trendy, black-rubber compacts, has become a favourite product among models and make-up professionals alike.

NARS' BACKSTAGE TRICKS OF THE TRADE

• Use translucent powder to tone down heavily-applied make-up and to blend eyeshadow.

• Always apply a lip treatment under lipstick: it makes the lips look more smooth.

• Use a powder puff instead of a brush because it helps powder to blend into the skin more easily.

• Never apply make-up to skin that hasn't been prepared with moisturiser and eye cream.

• Start with a small amount of colour – you can always add more but it's hard to remove after it has been applied.

• Never try to hide your true character – just transform yourself.

WHAT'S IN A MODEL'S MAKE-UP BAG

Mary Greenwell is to make-up what Bill Gates is to software: peek backstage at any show and you'll see her busily painting faces. Although she doesn't have her own signature line, Mary is the official make-up artist for, and adviser to, Elizabeth Arden. In order to give you a head start in achieving supermodel-style make-up, Mary has picked some of the items that she likes to work with, as well as the ones she's spotted in models' make-up bags.

BASE

Foundation: Bobbi Brown's Essentials Foundation Stick, Elizabeth Arden's Flawless-finish Mousse Make-up Foundation. **Tinted moisturiser:** Vichy's Tinted Moisturiser, Clarins' Tinted Moisturiser. **Powder:** Elizabeth Arden's Flawless Finish Loose Powder, Shu Uemura's Translucent Loose Powder. **Dual powder/foundation:** Lancôme's Maquilumine Compact, Dior's Teint Poudre. **Concealer:** Dior's Anticerne Perfecteur, Elizabeth Arden's Perfect Covering Concealer.

EYES

Eyeshadow: Elizabeth Arden's Eyeshadow Duo in Bare/Fawn. **For special effects:** Fardel's Maquillage Fluid Colours, Dior's Five-colour Eyeshadow Compact. **Mascara:** Elizabeth Arden's Two Brush Mascara. **Eyeliner:** Longcils' Boncza Liquid Eye Liner, Elizabeth Arden's Smoky Eyes Powder Pencil. **Brows:** YSL's Eyebrow Pencil.

LIPS

Liners: Elizabeth Arden's Lip Definer in Natural, Lancôme Le Stylo Contour des Lèvres in 05 Natural. **Lipsticks:** Chanel's Rouge à Lèvres in Rouge Pêche, Elizabeth Arden's Myth.

CHEEKS

Blush: Dior's Effets Blush Trio.

HIGHLIGHTER

Nars' The Multiple.

MAKE-UP ESSENTIALS

Aside from the make-up itself, models and make-up artists are never without those few indispensable items.

Q-tips (cotton buds) • Cotton balls • Tweezerman's tweezers • Dusting Powder (Mary creates it in the Elizabeth Arden lab) • D.R. Harris' eye drops • Tweezerman's eyelash curlers • Elizabeth Arden's Make-up Remover • Elizabeth Arden's Eight Hour Cream • L'Occitane's Moisturising Body Milk • A set of make-up brushes from ScreenFace.

STAR-QUALITY HAIRSTYLES

Celebrities and models all have one thing in common – a gorgeous head of hair.
Nicky Clarke – the celebrity hairdresser – and superstylist Guido present three different
looks so that you, too, can have superstar hair.

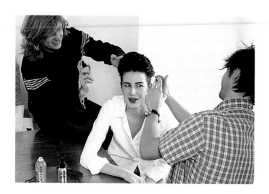

Nicky Clarke (left in picture above), with his Mayfair salon, VIP room and three-month waiting list, is hairdresser to the stars: Patsy Kensit, Liz Hurley, Gwyneth Paltrow, David Bowie, Andie MacDowell and Jemima Khan, to name but a few. He recently collaborated with the cutting-edge stylist Guido to create several modern hairstyles that have a touch of Nicky's coiffed look mixed with Guido's minimalist feel. 'Modern yet glamorous,' is how Nicky defines the three hairstyles featured here. 'The great thing about these styles is that as well as being classics, they are extremely versatile,' explains Nicky's creative director, Andrew Clark.

To sport a star-quality hairstyle á la Jennifer Aniston, Gwyneth Paltrow, et al, or to achieve one of Nicky and Guido's three looks, you need to follow these all important tips:

Tip 1 Get a good cut.

Tip 2 Rev up your hair's sheen with an excellent conditioner and regular treatments.

Tip 3 Equip yourself with the right styling tools, brushes and hairstyling products.

LOOK 1: THE MODERN SET

With this look, Nicky and Guido have created a modern take on a 'big-hair' classic. It has all the glamour created by root lift and body, but the straight ends and swept-back look give it a modern twist. Andrew tells you how to achieve it:

Step 1 Blast your hair with a hairdryer until it is about eighty per cent dry, blow-drying it to create volume by sweeping it in the opposite direction to which it naturally falls.

Step 2 Tip your head upside down and spritz the roots with a volumising product like Nicky's Hairomatherapy Lift, Thicken and Shine Spray.

Step 3 Take sections of hair from the front (approximately two inches from the hairline), then wind the hair in a backwards direction around a few big Velcro rollers (about two inches in diameter). Leave in for ten minutes and then remove the rollers.

Step 4 Brush your hair through. If you find that the ends are flicking up, flaten them by running straightening irons through your hair – swiftly so as not to cause damage.

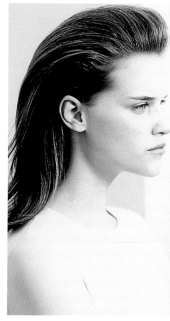

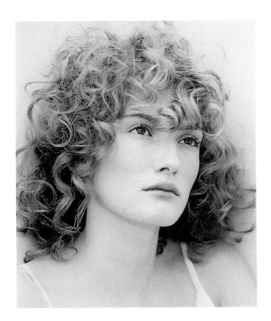

LOOK 2: CURLS

This is a relaxed, up-to-date version of a timeless look. By coaxing and separating the curls, this style gives a modern feel to naturally curly hair. Even if you haven't been blessed with a mop of curls, you can achieve this look from scratch with curling tools and a bit of patience. But take note – as Andrew points out, not all types of hair will curl or stay curly: 'The best hair to curl is very fine hair. Hair that is too straight or too heavy will drop quickly.'

For those with naturally curly hair

Step 1 Shampoo and condition your hair with products designed for curly hair as other preparations may add weight.

Step 2 To increase the hair's natural volume, tip your head upside down and blast your hair with a hairdryer until it is almost dry. Do not scrunch.

Step 3 Spray a little serum over the palms of both hands, then smooth a fine layer of it over your hair. If you are using liquid serum, rub your hands together to emulsify the serum before applying it to your hair. If you prefer, you can use mousse or wax.

Step 4 Tease and loosen your curls. Each natural curl should be separated three times.

For those who want to create curls from scratch

There are various types of curling tools available, but probably the speediest method of curling your hair is by using bendy sticks or the heated variety, such as Nicky's own brand Flexi Stylers; curling tongs work, but take longer.

Step 1 Shampoo and condition your hair. When it is nearly dry, take a chunk at a time and spray it with a holding product before winding it around a bendy stick. (Remember: the smaller the section, the smaller the curl.) Leave in for ten minutes or until hair is completely cool.

Step 2 Remove the bendy sticks and apply serum (see step 3, left).

Step 3 Tweak, tease and run your hands through your hair. The more tousled it looks, the better.

LOOK 3: TEXTURED BOB

'Sexy and tousled', says Nicky about this decidedly stylish, textured version of a basic bob. With choppy layers having been cut into it to add shape, the hair is then swept forward, which has a softening and flattering effect on the face. Playing devil's advocate, however, Andrew says that there's no point in torturing yourself by trying to get your hair to fall in a direction that it doesn't want to: 'If you are unsure as to which direction your hair naturally falls, ask your hairdresser,' he stresses. It is also essential to remember that good-looking short hair depends on the cut, so if you are 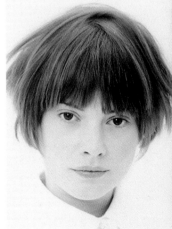 going for the chop, find the very best hairdresser.

Step 1 Starting off with damp hair, blast with a hairdryer until it is about eighty per cent dry, then spritz with a styling spray.

Step 2 Finish blow-drying brushing it forward.

Step 3 For the final touch, add a little serum (see step 3 of Look 2), and tousle.

HAIRCARE

Lustrous locks with body and bounce that swing as you
walk are your crowning glory. Here's how to get your mop in tiptop condition.

Colouring, perming, sunlight, heated styling aids and backcombing are just a few of the hair offenders that can turn glossy locks into dull, lacklustre, limp, frizzy or just difficult-to-manage hair – resulting in a bad-hair day every day. But there's no need to shy away from taking advantage of styling aids or the colourist's palette: 'virgin' hair is unquestionably the healthiest yet not necessarily the most beautiful. Even Philip Kingsley, the world's number one trichologist and author of *Hair* (Aurum, 1995), who has treated the likes of Ivana Trump, promotes hair colour and styling products as being great morale-boosters. If you look after your locks, you can counteract any damaging effects and still have beautiful tresses.

PHILIP KINGSLEY DISPELS THE HAIR MYTHS

Myth 1: brushing is good for your hair
It's not: overzealous brushing can damage your hair (try brushing a wool sweater and you'll soon see how quickly it wears out). Use your brush for styling only, and choose one that is made of plastic, not natural bristle or metal.

Myth 2: styling products damage your hair
Rubbish: styling products add shine and softness to your hair.

Myth 3: split ends can be mended
No serum can mend split ends: all it can do is glue them together temporarily. There is only one cure for split ends – cut them off.

Myth 4: vegetable colours are a hundred per cent natural
Natural ingredients are also chemicals: the plant may be natural, but its colouring effect relies on the chemical reaction caused by sunlight and soil composition when it was growing. Some of the worst cases of colour mistakes have been made with henna – a so-called 'natural' dye!

Myth 5: frequent washing will dry out hair
Not true: it's not oil flow that controls your hair's dryness but its moisture levels. Shampooing regularly with the right product, not a cheap, detergent shampoo, actually remoisturises hair.

Myth 6: cutting hair will make it grow stronger and faster
Cutting off the ends enhances thickness but will not affect your hair's actual growth.

Myth 7: too much conditioner will overcondition your hair
There is no such thing as overconditioning, in the same way that there is no such thing as being too healthy. If your hair looks limp and lifeless after conditioning it is either because you are using the wrong product, or because you have not rinsed it thoroughly.

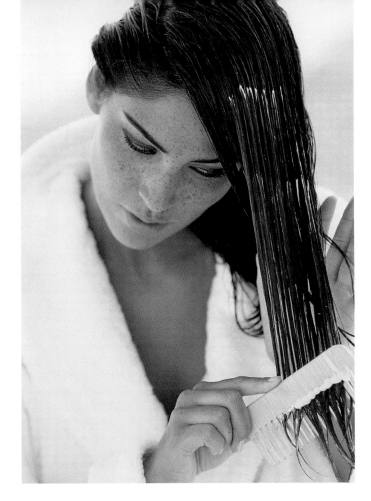

What is healthy hair and how can you achieve it?

Some shiny tresses give the illusion of healthy hair but, as Philip points out, because shine can be obtained with styling products, it is not necessarily a barometer of hair health. When hair is healthy, the cuticles lie flat and reflect the light, which leaves the hair with a natural sheen.

Hair grows on average half an inch a month – faster in summer. Naturally tough, healthy hair can expand by thirty per cent in length without breaking. And even after all the damaging things that we do to it – teasing, backcombing, colouring and blasting it with heat – it still remains resilient to a certain extent.

Hair is also incredibly responsive: by shampooing and conditioning it we can increase its moisture levels and make it stronger. Having your hair trimmed every four to six weeks will also keep your crowning glory in A1 condition. However, it doesn't matter how much conditioner you pile on if you don't nourish your hair from within. According to Philip, many people have lacklustre hair because of poor nutrition. The hair follicle is fed by a supply of blood, which should be crammed with nutrients, so eat a well-balanced diet, including plenty of fresh fruit and vegetables, and sufficient protein for amino acids. Take a vitamin-and-mineral supplement if you feel it necessary. (Vitamins and minerals known for their health-giving benefits to hair include vitamins A, B complex, C and E, iron, iodine, zinc and selenium.)

Assessing your hair type

Hair is often somewhat 'schizophrenic' – oily at the roots, yet lacking moisture at the ends – so make sure that you are not exacerbating the problem by, for example, using a shampoo for oily hair which will dry out the ends further. The way to assess your type is not by ascertaining whether it's oily, dry or normal. 'Assess your hair by its texture – fine, medium or thick – and whether the shape is straight, wavy, curly or frizzy', stresses Philip. 'And bear in mind that colour-treated or permed hair will always need more moisturising than "virgin" hair.'

Flaky scalp/dandruff

White flakes falling from your hair spoil even the most coiffed hair-do. Triggered off by such factors as poor diet and stress, both dandruff or a flaky scalp can be treated with a little care and attention: use a gentle, anti-dandruff shampoo until the condition clears up. (Philip suggests alternating this with your usual shampoo.) Because overusing an anti-dandruff shampoo can aggravate some hair problems and dehydrate your hair, once cured, switch back to your regular shampoo. You could also try cutting down on your intake of salty and spicy foods. Having attacked it from the inside out, if the condition still doesn't clear up, as it might be the result of seborrhoea dermatitis or psoriasis, you should seek the advise of a trichologist.

Shampooing

Philip strongly believes that shampooing is the most important aspect of hair health: firstly, because it replenishes moisturise; and, secondly, because it keeps hair tangle-free and washes away any dirt or grime. 'Your hair looks at its best when it is freshly washed, so I advise shampooing daily. You wouldn't go without showering', says Philip, with a smile. When shampooing your hair, don't forget to spend a couple of minutes massaging your scalp (either with your fingers or a scalp brush), as this increases blood flow to the scalp which, in turn, nourishes the hair follicle. Use this time to wash your brushes and combs, in order to prevent combing grime back into clean hair.

Here are a few of the good shampoos on the market: Al'chemey's Unscented Very Gentle Shampoo, J F Lazartigue's Shampoo for Dry Hair, Philip Kingsley's Body Building Shampoo, Phytologie's Phytomixte, Paul Mitchell's Shampoo 3, Garnier's Nutralia Healthy Hair Shampoo and Aussie's Moist Shampoo.

Conditioning

Whether it is short, long, fine, 'virgin', chemically treated or even oily, every head of hair needs some form of conditioner. A good conditioner untangles hair, smoothes the cuticles and replaces lost moisture. Pro-vitamin B5, humecterants and other state-of-the-art ingredients that are contained in many of today's products can actually penetrate the hair shaft and lock in moisture.

On the bottles of many conditioners you'll find instructions to the effect that you should leave the product on your hair for a certain length of time, but Philip says that this is not necessary: 'Any well-formulated conditioner should not need time to be effective. Besides, if left on too long it will dull the hair. Only treatments need time to work'. Speaking of which, Philip's advice is that all types and lengths of hair need regular treatments: 'If it's long, you need a treatment once a week, while short hair only needs it every month.' For your hair to really benefit, wrap your treated tresses in a warm towel or, even better, sit in a steam room or sauna.

Try one of the following treatments or conditioners: Philosophy's The Breaking Point, Philip Kingsley's Elasticizer, The Body Shop's Banana Hair Putty, Vidal Sassoon's Treatments Hair Moisturising Cream, Potion 9 by Sebastian, Kerastase's Masquintense, Redken's Climatress Moisturising Treatment, VO5's Hair Food or Charles Worthington's Results Hair Healer.

Care when drying

When your hair is wet, always use a comb, not a brush, to remove tangles. Start at the ends and gently work upwards. If you come across a nasty tangle, spritz it with a little leave-in conditioner; the comb should glide through easily. Do not rub your hair with a towel: this roughens up cuticles and deprives the hair of its natural shine. Rather than blasting your hair with heat, allow it to dry naturally until it is about eighty per cent dry and only then reach for the hairdryer. Shield your hair from the heat by spraying it with a protective product, such as Neutrogena's Heat Safe or Paul Mitchell's The Heat.

Handling heated styling aids

Labelled 'the tools of destruction' by Philip, heated rollers, straightening irons, hot brushes or other metal appliances can seriously damage hair if not used correctly, leaving you with dry, brittle and even singed hair that splits and breaks easily. Do not allow heated appliances to get too hot and remember that the metal types, like tongs and straightening irons, are your hair's arch-enemies. You wouldn't dream of running your clothes iron over your hair, so you'd be wise to take extreme care when using metal styling aids. Hold any heated appliance in the hair for only the minimum amount of time and guard hair with a protective product.

Perms

Popular in the 1970s and early 1980s, perms have been now superseded by colour in fashion terms. Even when curls rule the runways, a perm is too 'permanent' to change with the diktat of hair fashion – no sooner will you have mastered how to tousle your perm when curls will be passé. Stick to tongs or curlers. If you still want to take the plunge, the good news is that today's acid perms are far more sophisticated than perming solutions used to be. However, as a perm alters the hair's structure, it is a harsh process that cannot be reversed and that does not work well with colour; there is also the added problem of regrowth. If your hair is permed, you need to take extra care when looking after it and should only use products that are specially formulated for permed or chemically treated hair.

Sunproof hair

Sunshine alone will bleach and dehydrate your locks, penetrating the hair shaft and causing hair to become brittle and lifeless, but add to that the drying effects of sea salt, sand and chlorinated swimming-pools, and you have a lethal mix that will take more than an intensive treatment to remedy. What's worse, if your hair is tinted or highlighted, you could return from your holiday sporting a green- or orange-tinged head of hair to complement your tan!

In order to protect your hair from the elements, before sunbathing or swimming spray or comb in a sun-, or sun-and-swim-protection product, but remember that there's nothing quite as effective as covering your hair with a hat or bandanna when sunbathing. Don't forget to protect your scalp, too, and always shampoo your hair after swimming.

Try Phytoplage's High Protection Sun Oil, J F Lazartigue's Protective Oil for Hair, Bumble and Bumble's Sun Spray, Schwarzkopf's Bona-Cure Suncare Sun Protection Spray and Philip Kingsley's Swimcap Cream.

Hair loss and thinning hair

The average number of hairs on each head is 120,000. We all lose up to a hundred hairs a day, but chronic hair loss (known as alopecia), which causes thinning or a receding hairline, can be a traumatic experience – especially for women. At the first sign of hair loss you should consult a trichologist.

Philip emphasises that the reasons for hair loss are complex: hormones, stress, anaemia, poor diet, pregnancy and genetic factors are just some of the triggers. 'Once the reasons have been discovered, plenty can be done to alleviate the problem,' says Philip, although he points out that it's no good just rubbing potions on your head or popping pills in the vain hope that they will bring your hair back.

Cosmetically, hair that is thinning can be dramatically improved in appearance with hair extensions. Even in cases of severe hair loss or balding, we no longer have to resort to a wig or toupee, for according to dermatologist Professor Nicholas Lowe, there are now successful hair transplants: 'We take tiny micrografts of skin from the back of the scalp and graft them onto the area of hair loss, which is normally at the front. The hair grows back naturally again shortly after the operation.'

REINVENT YOURSELF WITH COLOUR

Hair without colour is like a face without make-up: it looks bare and undressed.
So whether you want to brighten up lacklustre hair or totally reinvent yourself, colour is the
must-have hair accessory that no woman should be without.

Hair colour lifts your whole appearance, revives jaded hair and is one of the most effective beautifiers. 'With the latest technology and superior formulations, colour has never been easier', says Jo Hansford, the queen of colour who has a star-studded clientele. At Jo's exclusive Mayfair salon, you might find yourself sitting next to Carla Bruni, Melanie Griffith, Kate Winslet or another celebrity, which is exactly what happened to me when Jo performed her Midas touch on what I thought was an irreversible hair disaster. A few hours and a smattering of reverse lights and highlights later, I walked out with a mane that any celebrity would have been be proud of.

JO HANSFORD'S ADVICE ON PROFESSIONAL COLOURING

• Before colouring your hair, think about the upkeep involved and consider whether you can maintain the colour (in terms of both cost and time). Highlights need redoing approximately every three months and permanent tints every four weeks.
• When choosing a colourist, find a salon with a colour technician (a hairdresser who specializes in colour) – rather than a general hairdresser who is a jack of all trades.
• A good hairdresser should give you a consultation and advise you against a colour if he or she doesn't think that it will work or suite you for that matter.
• Ask the colourist first to test your chosen colour on small piece of your hair and then live with it for a couple of days before deciding if it's really what you want.

QUESTIONS AND ANSWERS

Will colour damage my hair?

Hair colour has come on in leaps and bounds in the past few years and cotton-wool-like hair and green tinges are now things of the past. As so long as it is applied by a qualified hairdresser who is experienced in colouring, the process will not damage your hair. In fact, colour can improve the texture of your hair, for it adds body to fine or limp hair, and depth and shine to dull hair.

How can I maintain my colour or retouch my roots between salon visits?

If your hair colour has faded, vegetable colours, colour mousses or colour-enhancing shampoos and conditioners, will liven it up. For those who lighten their hair and hence suffer from regrowth, Jo's tip for defusing the darkness of the roots is to apply a tiny amount of dry-shampoo powder along the parting, dusting off any excess. Alternatively, you could try using a hair colour-mascara wand, such as Dior's Mascara Flash for Hair.

My hair colour is a disaster – is there anything that can be done to rectify it?

According to Jo, with the exception of henna colours (which are virtually impossible to colour over), most colour disasters can be remedied. Jo recalls being faced with a Spanish model whose lime-green-tinged, straw-like hair needed to look fabulous (for a hair advertisement, no less) in a matter of hours. Jo succeeded.

How should I care for coloured hair?

Keep your hair out of the sun because it can fade the colour through oxidation. Use shampoos and conditioners that have been specially formulated for coloured hair and apply a weekly intensive-conditioning treatment.

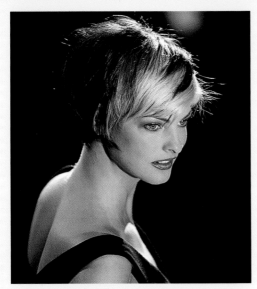

Colour chameleon Linda Evangelista reinvents herself with colour.

THE COLOUR GUIDE

Here is a list of the different types of colouring products and techniques currently available.

Mascara wands, powder and colour mousses are great inventions: you can add colour or streaks to match your outfit, or brush on shimmer with a powder, such as Dior's Highlighting Powder For Hair, and then wash out the following day.

Colour-enhancing shampoos and conditioners: by coating the hair's cuticles, these products enhance your hair colour and keep coloured hair vibrant. To avoid build-up, Jo advises against using them continuously.

Semi-permanent colours coat the surface of the hair for six to eight washes and are great for enhancing your natural colour with such shades as chestnut, warm reds and gold tones.

Tone-on-tone/demi-permanent colours are hair colours that last for up to twenty washes and contain no ammonia, only low levels of chemicals which permeate the outer cortex and coat the cuticle. They are suitable if you want a richer or darker shade, but won't lighten your hair. Do not use on hair that has been highlighted or tinted.

Vegetable dyes can enrich, deepen the shade or tone down brassy hair colour. As they only coat the hair, vegetable colours wash out after approximately six to eight washes, although this depends on the length of time the dye has been left on the hair.

Henna: avoid henna like the plague, unless you want to risk going green.

Tints/permanent colours contain ammonia and peroxide. Because they do not wash out, the roots need redoing every four weeks.

Highlights use permanent tint – of one or more shades – to lighten the hair and are either woven in in ultra-fine sections for a subtle effect, or are applied in chunky slices for more noticeable results. Can also be introduced around the face for a sunkissed look.

Lowlights are applied using the same method as highlights but are of darker shades, such as golden browns and reds, rather than blonde tones.

Reverse lights use a tint – often similar to the client's natural colour – to break up areas of solid dye.

How do I choose the right colour?

The majority of people arrive at the salon knowing what they want but, according to Jo, a hairdresser is more skilled and experienced to judge the colour that will flatter the clients skin tone, than the client. In general, blonde shades suit most skin tones, but those with olive skin should avoid the lighter shades. Red tones are more tricky and do not suit those with pinkish colouring. And, whereas brunette shades suit most, raven hair can make some people look pallid and washed out.

Can I colour my hair at home?

Doing it yourself may save money in the short term, but unless you are using a wash-in-wash-out formula it can be risky: 'Most women end up coming to a salon to correct home horrors', says Jo. For fool-proof results, Jo, who has her own range of hair colour, Couture Colour, suggests that you read the instructions of any hair dye twice and carry out a strand test first. If a product has taken more strongly than you expected, Jo has a DIY tip to help soften the colour: 'Soak your hair for one hour in olive oil – this will soften the cuticles and release some of the colour.' Permanent tints, highlights and lowlights should be left to the professionals.

READY-TO-WEAR HAIRSTYLING

Modern hairstyles are easy to wear and effortless to achieve. Equipped with the right tools, styling products and experts' tricks of the trade, you can look like you've just stepped out of the salon.

THE RIGHT HAIRCUT

Nothing looks quite as good as a sharp, new haircut, and once your hair has been cut into a distinctive style, home maintenance becomes effortless. Before you take the plunge with a new hairstyle, however, make sure that your hairdresser explains its upkeep and the approximate styling time that it will take in order to recreate the look at home. Maintain the shape of your style by having your hair trimmed every four to six weeks – this way it is less likely to behave temperamentally.

Remember that the most successful hairstyles work well when they suit the hair type. Desperately trying to dry your Pre-Raphaelite curls poker-straight every day will cause you endless frustration, damage your hair and make you late for work. It's pointless having a salon 'do' that takes hours to style when all you want to do each day is wash 'n' go!

A GUIDE TO STYLING PRODUCTS

Confused by the labyrinth of rows upon rows of styling products? Here's a guide to the different types of styling products currently available and a run-down on the looks that each can achieve.

Mousse defines curl and boosts the volume of fine, fly-away hair.

Serum/silicone smooths, imparts shine, improves condition, defrizzes and controls fly-away hair.

Styling spray thickens, boosts volume, straightens, aids styling and holds hair in place.

Gel is most suitable for sculpting and holding a short hairstyle. Some straightening products also come in gel form.

Wax smoothes and tames hair and is often used to give hair a wet, slicked-back look. Pomades and grooming creams achieve similar results.

Hair-protectors shield hair from the damage caused by blow-drying and heated appliances.

Hairspray holds hair in place but, too much of the stuff and you'll end up with hair as stiff as cardboard. However, for styles that easily lose their shape, a light misting of hairspray once the hair is dry will help hold the style for longer.

Products John Frieda's Frizz Ease, Nicky Clarke's Hairomatherapy Lift, Thicken and Shine Spray, Schwarzkopf's Supersoft Vitamin Complex Hairspray, Phytologie's Phytovolume Actif, Oribe's Pomade, Sam McKnight's Definitive Style Starter, Salon Selective's Alcohol-free Nourishing Styling Mousse, Tigi's Pure-gloss Finishing, Philosophy's Let's Get Something Straight, Sebastian's Laminates Hi Gloss Drops and Joico's Spray Gel.

TOOLS OF THE TRADE

Blow-dryers should have three heat settings (including a cool setting) and two speeds. To avoid frying hair, hold the hairdryer at least six inches away from your hair and, on the medium or cool setting, rough-dry your hair until it is about eighty per cent dry before you attempt to style it (make sure that you keep the air stream moving). Now style your hair with a brush until it is completely dry. (If your hair is slightly damp the style will drop, but take care that you don't overdry it.)

Diffuser attachments disperse the air through little jets and are great for preventing frizz and introducing root lift when used on curly hair.

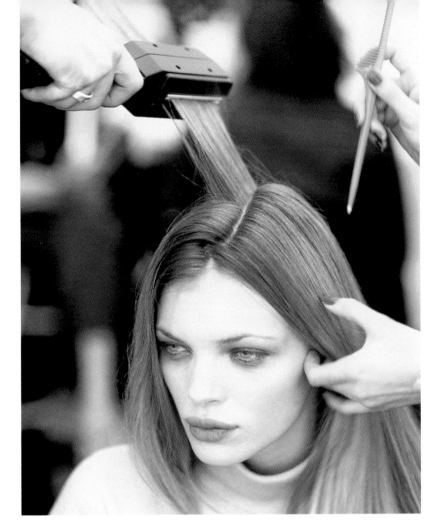

Blow-dryers with built-in stylers blow out a jet of hot air and are useful for adding volume and flipping up or curling under ends.

Straightening irons and crimpers have heated metal plates that either iron out any waves and kinks or, using a crimped-iron attachment, add lots of little waves to the hair. To avoid damage, run the iron swiftly through the hair or hold it for the minimum amount of time. You can also use these tools to crimp or straighten the loose ends of 'hair-up-dos'.

Curling tongs are useful as a quick fix, to flip up or curl under ends, or to curl the tendrils around your face when wearing hair up.

Hot brushes achieve a similar affect to tongs, but their wands are covered in brush-like spikes.

Heated rollers are useful if you want to create various size curls or volume at the roots and crown. However, they can damage your hair, so if you own the traditional, plastic spiked type, place a piece of tissue around each roller before winding your hair round it. Even better, buy the more hair-friendly rubber or steam rollers.

Velcro rollers are favoured by many hairstylists. They are self-grip, come in all sizes and do not damage the hair with heat. Use them to achieve volume or curl; a couple of extra-large ones will help smooth out and straighten your hair.

Bendy sticks are the modern-day equivalent of rags (you can also buy them in heated form) and can be used to create curls or a head of waves. Divide your hair into small sections and then simply wind the hair around them, twisting the ends of the sticks to secure.

Brushes popular for salon-type styling include the round, barrel brush, a paddle brush and a vent brush. Brushes can also be used for teasing the hair and backcombing it at the roots to give lift and volume.

Combs are favoured for grooming and for use on wet hair as they cause less damage than a brush. A small-toothed comb is useful for backcombing, while the wide-toothed type is suitable for untangling wet hair and taming curly hair.

CREATING VOLUME

Unless you wear your hair in a style that is close to your head, you will probably want to create volume and lift at the roots. According to celebrity hairdresser Nicky Clarke, your haircut is important in achieving this: 'Layering can give your hair instant volume if done well,' says the man who is synonymous with volume. Here are Nicky's tips for creating lift and fullness at home.

Step 1 While your hair is wet, tip your head upside down or sweep your hair in the opposite direction to that which it naturally lies and blow-dry, directing the heat at the roots and shaping the hair with a large, round, bristle brush.

Step 2 When your hair is about eighty per cent dry, wind a few large Velcro rollers into the hair at the crown, spray them with a volumising lotion and blow-dry until your hair is completely dry (hair drops if it's the slightest bit damp).

Step 3 Leave them for ten minutes, then remove the rollers and tease your hair into place.

GET SHINY

Whether it's sleek or tousled, most of us want that supermodel sheen. Nicky Clarke's creative director, Andrew Clark, stresses that over applying styling and shine-enhancing products, as well as leave-in conditioners, can make hair look lank and lacklustre: 'Always use a small amount of the product to begin with', he says, continuing 'Serum is a brilliant product, for instance, but if you over do it, your only option will be to wash your hair and start all over again. Whether it's spray or liquid serum, apply to hands first before smoothing onto hair. This way you are more likely to distribute it evenly.' Here's how to get shine the Nicky Clarke way.

Step 1 Shampoo and condition your hair with products that are suited to it.

Step 2 Rinse your hair thoroughly.

Step 3 Resist rubbing your hair with a towel: the rubbing action raises the cuticles and prevents any possibility of having shiny hair.

Step 4 Blow-dry your hair, brushing it from the roots to the ends and pointing the blow-dryer downwards so that the hair's cuticles lie flat.

Step 5 When your hair is nearly dry, smooth on a shine-promoting product such as Nicky's Hairomatherapy Spray and Shine Serum (a good product not only coats the hair cosmetically but also helps to seal the cuticles).

HOW TO HAVE SMOOTH, SLEEK STRAIGHT HAIR

Few of us are born with sleek, poker straight hair, but it is a look that many of us struggle to achieve. Here style supremo Kevin Mancuso, author of *The Mane Thing* (Alias Books, 1998), tells you how to straighten your hair so it is as smooth as glass – and keep it that way.

Step 1 First, apply a straightening gel to the hair, working from the roots to the ends. Then, if you like, add a small amount of grooming cream, serum or a silicone product to the ends and outer layer of the hair only, to give added straightness, shine and control.

Step 2 Using a flat, boar-bristle brush and your blow-dryer (with the compression nozzle in place), gently pull your hair down from underneath while directing the air flow onto, not into, your hair.

Step 3 When you have finished drying your hair, adding a tiny bit more grooming cream, serum or silicone will add shine and control any flyaway tendencies.

HOW TO AVOID A SALON DISASTER

You walked into the salon with high hopes of looking like a million dollars but left in floods of tears. Here are some tips from Ian Denson, the creative director of the internationally renowned hairdresser John Frieda, to help you avoid a potential salon disaster.

- **Choosing the right salon:** How on earth do you decide which salon you can entrust your hair to? Ian suggests stalking out the place first: 'Get a cup of coffee and sit outside the salon for half an hour or so and check out the hair-dos of clients leaving. Ask yourself "Is the salon busy and do the people leaving it look good?"' Ian also suggests that asking for recommendations from friends, or seeing which magazines endorse which salons, are other useful methods of finding a good hairdresser. And, if you happen to spot a woman sporting that to-die-for hairstyle that you've always wanted, why not stop her and ask her where she had her hair done.

- **Insist on a consultation:** 'If a hairdresser hasn't got time for a consultation, walk out,' insists Ian. 'If the stylist says "leave it to me", don't. A hairstylist should never insist on cutting your hair in a certain way unless you agree to it. Don't forget: you are the one who has to live with it.' Note that all stylists should consult you while your hair is still dry in order for them to assess the true colour and texture of your hair.

- **Communicate:** Many people leave a salon feeling disappointed because they have not told their stylist precisely what they want. Discuss with your stylist exactly the style you are after, as well as what you definitely don't want. 'It's no good telling the hairdresser that you still want to be able to wear your hair up in a chignon when he's halfway through cutting it short,' says Ian, speaking from experience. 'Never think that you are hassling the hairdresser. If you walk away content, the chances are that the salon will have secured your custom.'

- **Take a picture along:** If you have a definite idea of the hairstyle you want, a photograph or two can help the stylist. 'A picture is a good idea as long as you use it for inspiration only,' stresses Ian. 'The person in the photo is likely to have different-textured hair. Also, a picture is static and only shows the front of the hairstyle. People tend to forget that their hair can be seen from 360°.' Any decent stylist should tell you how the hairstyle in your picture can be adapted and tailored to suit you. But be prepared for the stylist to advise you against it: it's no good pleading for the 'Rachel' cut if you've got coarse, wavy hair (even if it is *the* most copied style).

- **Utilise your hairdresser's expertise:** Stylists work with hair every day and are therefore a great source of advice. Most will be more than willing to advise you on such things as home-grooming, different ways in which to wear your tresses, which products to use and how to care for and manage your style. Ian's tip is to take along a bag of products and styling tools to show your hairdresser exactly what you work with at home.

- **Listen to suggestions:** Stylists are experts on hair and can advise you on those haircuts that both suit your face shape and work well with your hair's texture. A good hairdresser should take all sorts of factors into account before reaching for the scissors or deciding on a colour solution. 'I look at my client's height, frame, build and whether or not they have confidence', explains Ian. 'We discuss things like lifestyle, work and how much time they have to do their hair each morning.'

- **Don't make a rash decision:** Having to live with a bad hair decision is not the end of the world, but it can be depressing and lower your self-confidence, so don't be hasty: take your time and ponder the pros and cons of a new style before taking the plunge.

CATWALK-STYLE HAIR

A touch daring, a little bit sexy and utterly creative – catwalk-style hair will vamp up your image. All it takes is a little imagination and a few accessories to look like you are a regular on the runway.

MAKING A STATEMENT

Catwalk-style hair is not for the intrepid but for those who want to make a statement. Far from being practical, and like the often outlandish designer clothes we see regularly paraded down the runway, show hair represents creation without limits: it's over the top, dramatic and often ridiculous, 'hair-raising' stuff. Not surprisingly, runway hairstyles have become almost as headline-grabbing as the clothes, and many a supermodel has been catapulted to superstardom thanks to her catwalk hair-do.

If you have seen any runway shots or footage from the shows with the more outrageous hair-dos, you're probably thinking that you wouldn't want to be seen dead with a bottle-green crop, metal spikes poking out of your hair or a feathered Mohican that looks more like a stuffed animal balanced on top of your head. But, according to innovator of hair trends and catwalk-hair maestro Sam McKnight, it is not all so over the top: 'At Antonio Baradi, hair was outrageous, yet the same season, at Paul Smith, it was simple and unconstructed,' says Sam, who created the hairstyles for both shows.

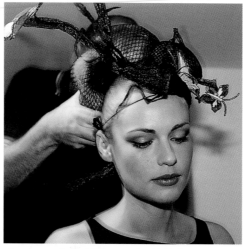

'Relaxed', 'easy' and 'effortless' are the buzz words for modern catwalk-style hair: 'The key is to not look like you've tried too hard,' says Sam, who, before deciding on the hairstyle, always takes the clothes into consideration first. 'It's essential that there is a theme running through the clothes and hair', he says. 'This is what you should aim to create at home – not a hairstyle and an outfit, but a total look.' Before you reach for the styling brush, a versatile, precision cut by a good stylist is a vital prerequisite for catwalk-style hair. And, it goes with out saying that your tresses should be in tip top condition, so start treating them now.

ELEMENTS OF CATWALK HAIR

There are certain elements of catwalk hair that work extremely well off the runway. Featured here are the main components that grace the runways season after season. So be creative and customise your hair for a stunning, catwalk-style look that is unique to you.

Prepare your hair

Sam explains how important it is to prepare your hair for a catwalk style: 'Freshly washed hair is the most difficult to style as it is flyaway, slippery and often unmanageable. The moment I sit a model down, I prime her hair with a product that I developed as a style-starter, so the hair behaves better.' Before you start working on your creation, use some form of styling product; Sam suggests making your own customised styling product by mixing mousse and gel, or mousse and wax, for example. Depending on your hair type, sometimes you need to use one product on the roots and a different one on the hair itself. You only ever need a tiny amount. And always go easy to begin with: you can add more if required. Don't worry about styling products clinging to the hair – they all wash out if you rinse well.

Adorn your hair with accessories

By adorning your hair with decorative butterflies, feathers and flowers (real and fake), ribbons, scarves, bands, clips, slides, tiaras or even the letters of the alphabet, you can create your own individual hairstyle. But keep it simple: a single feather or a strategically placed Alice band (see picture of Kirsty Hume right), is all you need.

You'll find hair accessories in fashion boutiques, accessory shops and department stores, but for the more unusual piece you may want to head off the beaten track. Sam scours all sorts of places, from haberdashery and bead shops to antique shops for old silk flowers, as well as gardening shops for raffia. 'Keep your eye open for the unusual. I have stumbled across such goodies as little holographic stars and glass flowers', enthuses Sam. 'You could also do as I do and make your own hair accessories.' One of Sam's most innovative show-hair accessories was for a Matthew Williamson show (see picture on opposite page): 'I stuffed neon-coloured hairpieces into black fishnet tights and then used them to make classic chignons.' Try this one at home!

Become colour crazy

Whether it be two-tone hair, bold, skunk-like, fiery stripes or neon-coloured slices, runway colour is often intentionally fake, as it is these bolts of brilliance that make any head of hair show-worthy. But you don't need to dye your hair: use colour mousses, hair mascara or hair powder.

Another simple way in which to achieve catwalk colour is to attach coloured hairpieces to your hair or to use sprays in eye-catching reds, golds and silvers. This way you can create dramatic colour contrasts without damaging your hair. To customise your own hairpiece, Sam suggests dying it yourself.

Catwalk braids and ponytails

Play around with your hair: braid it in different ways or pull it back into a ponytail, letting a few tendrils slip out here and there. Utilise your own hair: secure a section of hair into a ponytail, leaving two chunks loose on either side and then wind these remaining sections around the elastic, tuck under the ends, and secure them with a grip. Alternatively, sweep hair back securing part of the hair just below your crown in a band. Now wind a band around the remainder of your hair at the nape of your neck.

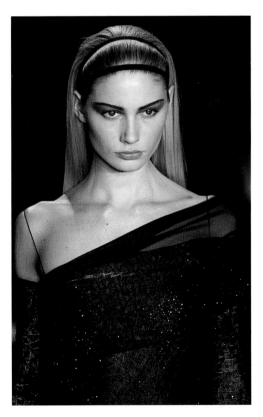

Party hair decorated with beads

Party time demands that extra-special hair-do and is the definitely the occasion when catwalk-style hair works best. One hair-do that you can easily recreate is the beaded chignon: simply take strands of beads and wind them around the elastic of your chignon or ponytail. Another easy look can be created by sprinkling beads over slicked-back hair; you can buy individual beads or, if you have an inexpensive or old necklace, split it up and use some of its beads. Glitter and sequins also work well. For this look, Sam suggests sweeping back your hair into a messy topknot or ponytail first: 'Spread a little eyelash glue over the parts of hair that you want to decorate; eyelash glue is easy to peel off and will not damage your hair. Then, either strategically place the beads or sprinkle them over the glue.'

Transform yourself with a hairpiece

Clip on a false bang, add an instant, low-slung ponytail, or slide in a teddy-boy-style quiff to transform yourself in a matter of minutes. Sam tells you how: 'You can make your own hairpiece by buying the hair, then sewing it onto a little comb. To apply the hairpiece, lift your hair up from under the parting, take a clump of hair and backcomb it at the roots. Then slide the hairpiece into the backcombed roots.'

Wacky wigs

Have you ever wondered how models magically transform their hair from short to long and from blonde to red at a click of a camera's shutter? The answer lies in a wig. Ranging from real-hair wigs that will match your natural colour to crazily coloured synthetic ones, wigs are very sophisticated these days. It's well worth having your wig fixed professionally at first, so that when you are faced with putting it on it at home for the first time you get it right – there's nothing quite so unglamorous as your wig flying down the high street! When buying a wig, remember that a half-wig, which is ideal for giving volume and length to hair, is easier to fix than a full wig. A final tip: once you've made your purchase, have your wig cut on your head – this way it can be styled to match your real hair and suit your face shape.

Bangs

A familiar sight on most catwalks, bangs (the new word for fringe) come in many different shapes and forms. The beauty of a bang is that it's versatile: wear it slicked back, feathered, clipped to one side or falling forward; you can also trim it yourself.

Sexy textures

Hair is often let loose on the catwalk, displaying a variety of textures: smooth and sleek, curly, wavy, kinked and crimped, or tousled for an unstructured look. To achieve different textures, use styling tools, such as Velcro rollers, bendy sticks, tongs, crimping and straightening irons, as well as styling products that thicken, add body and smooth the hair. You don't have to stick to the same texture all over. Take random pieces, leaving the rest of your hair natural.

Slicked-back hair

Models parading down the runway with slicked-back, wet-look hair inject sophistication into any show. This is one of the easiest catwalk looks to achieve, but watch out: on the wrong head it could end up looking like your hair hasn't seen shampoo for a month. It goes without saying that the slicked-back look works best on short hair. However, it can work on long hair if tied in a ponytail or swept back into a neat chignon.

Backcombing

For creating hair that is big and bouffant or to add lift at roots or crown, backcombing is guaranteed to give almost any hairstyle that coiffured, catwalk look. Using a brush or fine-toothed comb, backcomb your hair gently at the roots. Spritz it with hairspray to hold in place.

Unstructured hair

When catwalk hair isn't smooth, sleek or elaborate it is often teased and backcombed to look undone. Bird's-nest chic or just-got-out-of-bed-hair: some of the hairstyles have been positively deconstructed. You don't have to go mad with the backcombing and messing up to achieve an unstructured look – just tousle it a little and then let your hair do its own thing.

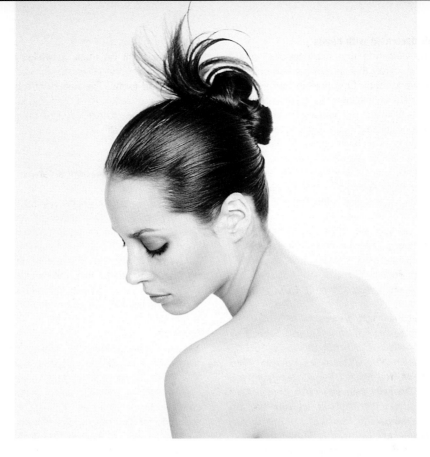

'HAIR UP-DOS'

The catwalk appears to have a continuous love affair with the 'up-do' – hair that is worn up. Piling your hair on your head is a clever way of looking like you've just stepped off the runway. The up-do comes in all shapes and sizes, but the key is not to let it look too overdone. Here are some different up-dos for you to try.

● **Quick and simple:** fasten your hair into a ponytail using a fabric-covered elastic somewhere between your crown and the nape of your neck. Having pulled your hair through the elastic once, the second time you bring the ponytail through stop halfway and secure it. If you want it to look less structured, tease out little bits of hair and curl, crimp or straighten, before applying a smidgen of gel, wax or serum with your fingers to separate the ends.

● **The twist and roll:** having spritzed your hair with styling lotion, sweep it back off your face into a ponytail at the nape of your neck. Now twist the ponytail towards the crown, roll in the ends and secure the ponytail with a couple of clips or pins.

● **The topknot:** pile your hair into a high ponytail at the top of your crown using a fabric-covered elastic. Wind the hair around the elastic and secure it with a clip (pull out a few strands if you like and add texture with styling aids).

● **A head of little twists:** separate your hair into several little bunches, then haphazardly twist and fold each section before pinning it to your head with kirby grips. Another desirable twist, which makes you look as though you have a head full of little topknots, is created by scrunching up each section into a little bundle and securing it with fabric-covered elastic.

HOLDING BACK THE YEARS

To hell with growing old gracefully – take advantage
of the latest weapons in the battle against ageing and stave off the wrinkles.

For years we've heard the same depressing message: 'You can't do anything to prevent or reverse ageing other than resorting to the knife'. Having always believed this to be absolute rubbish, when I hit the big 3-0 and realised that I was no longer immune to the forces of gravity, I dug out every scrap of research on ageing.

Anyone past thirty will know that ageing isn't just about getting wrinkles: it's also about half-a-dozen or so other age-related afflictions – under-eye bags, droopy eyelids, saggy and crepy skin, open pores and, as if all that wasn't depressing enough, jowls and a slackening jaw line. Ageing is an unstoppable force of nature and there are no miracle cures for it – yet. Nonetheless, with a little help you can rejuvenate your skin and guard against the ravages of time. But before we look at anti-ageing aids, it is important to realise that the mind is the most powerful anti-ager: stop worrying about your wrinkles and you will be well over halfway towards knocking years off your age.

SKIN PHYSIOLOGY

In order to be able to care for your skin properly you need to understand the skin's ageing process. So if you didn't pay attention in biology classes, here is a little basic information on skin physiology for you to digest.

The structure of the skin is made up of two main layers. The epidermis – the uppermost layer – is the visible part, which is constructed of a horny layer of skin containing the dead skin cells that we slough off during exfoliation. The second layer – the dermis, or 'true' skin – is composed of connective tissue: collagen and elastin fibres which, by keeping it resilient and springy, are the skin's support network. Within the dermis, you'll also find sebaceous glands (which secrete sebum, the skin's natural lubricant) and the blood vessels that supply vital nourishment and oxygen to the cells.

From our mid-twenties the time bandits set to work: the rate of cell renewal slows down, moisture levels drop and collagen production is reduced, causing loss of elasticity. Meanwhile, the production rate of line-forming free radicals – those nasty molecules that degenerate cells – speeds up and eventually the skin's muscle tone deteriorates and its support structure collapses.

How you age is, to a certain extent, determined by your genes, but before you blame your parents for frown lines so deep that only Polyfilla would disguise them, let me reassure you that this doesn't mean that you will age at the same rate as they did. We are now far more clued up on what we should and should not be doing to our skin than our parents' generation. And besides, each of us ages differently, so just because you are forty doesn't mean that you will have fifty per cent grey hair, five wrinkles on your forehead and a 'turkey neck' like your mother.

AGE DEFENCE IN A NUTSHELL

Dr Catherine Orentreich, a dermatologist at the world-famous Orentreich Medical Group LLP in New York, is one of the leading authorities on skin ageing. Being well acquainted with one of her patients, who at thirty-three has younger-looking skin than when she was in her teens, I decided that Dr Orentreich was the ideal person to advise on age-defence strategies.

Dr Orentreich believes in the traditional formula of cleansing, exfoliating and moisturising. She is also hot on protection: 'Everyone should

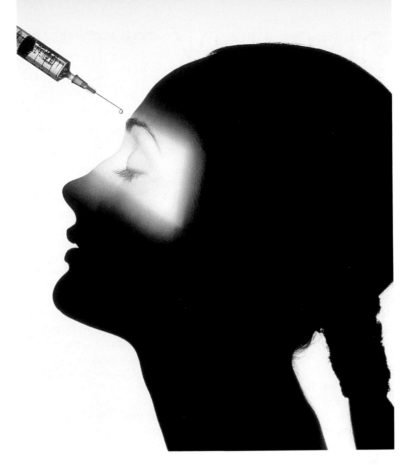

be wearing a sunblock on their face,' she adds. I asked Dr Orentreich how she would treat the skin of a woman in her thirties who is beginning to see signs of ageing. 'I might prescribe a Retin-A preparation, a "vitamin-A derivative" that improves the skin's texture, to be used as part of her skincare routine. In addition, a gentle skin peel, using trichloroacetic acid, could be carried out three to four times a year,' she advises.

ANTI-AGEING AIDS

Potions and lotions

Can we buy youth in a jar or is the advertising – with its promise to reconstruct the skin and make us look years younger – spurious? Vitamins A, C and E, co-enzyme Q10, Emu oil, Blue copper, enzymes, fat cell extracts and oxygen are just some of the anti-ageing ingredients currently being trumpeted by cosmetic companies. And while some will indeed continue to be the mainstay ingredients of anti-ageing products, others will be deemed ineffective after the hype dies down and the lab tests are exhausted. Dr Orentreich points out that even the new generation of anti-ageing moisturisers cannot reverse ageing by changing the structure of the skin. However, because these creams contain hydrating ingredients, she believes that they can improve the skin's ability to retain moisture which, in turn, temporarily plumps out wrinkles to give the complexion a smoother appearance.

With Crème De La Mer face cream being snapped up at $150 a jar, surely even the wealthiest beauty aficionados wouldn't fork out such silly money unless they saw some results, so here are a few of the better anti-ageing elixirs around, from ones costing only a few pounds to the most expensive: Nivea's Visage Anti-wrinkle Q10 Cream, L'Oréal's Plenitude Revitalift, Nina Ricci's Time Defense Extract, YSL's Prevention +, La Prairie's Cellular Complex Cream, Shiseido's Bio Performance Advanced Super-revitalizer Whitening Formula, Osmotic's Blue Copper Firming Elasticity Repair, Kanebo's Ex La Crème, Caudalie's Grape-seed Rejuvinating Cream and Crème De La Mer.

Cosmeceuticals

If you know your AHAs from your BHAs, you are probably familiar with the cosmeceutical. For those who aren't au fait with skincare jargon, the word was coined by Dr Albert Kligman, a leading authority on skin and a professor at the University of Pennsylvania. This label is given to anti-ageing products that are neither strictly topical drugs nor cosmetics, but lurk somewhere in the middle, containing as they do higher concentrates of active ingredients than their cosmetic counterparts. Retin-A, AHAs (Alpha-hydroxy acids), BHAs (Beta-hydroxy acids) and vitamin C are some the key ingredients found in such products.

AHAs and BHAs

Alpha-hydroxy acids, also known as fruit acids, were probably the most coveted ingredients in anti-ageing products in recent years. Lauded for their exfoliating action, they sparked off a craze in which almost every skincare range contained at least one AHA product.

Derived from lemon juice, sour milk, sugar cane, apples, grapes and red wine, the three main AHAs are glycolic, lactic and citric acid. AHAs slough off dead skin cells, causing living cells to divide more rapidly, and therefore stimulate cell metabolism. But Dr Orentreich stresses that AHAs can irritate the skin and for this reason prefers Beta-hydroxy acids as the less abrasive alternative for skin renewal: 'BHAs have many proven properties but, unlike AHAs, they are non-irritant and anti-inflammatory', she explains. The most widely used BHA is salicylic acid, which is derived from willow bark.

Topical vitamins and antioxidants

Antioxidant vitamins (A, C and E) neutralise the ageing effects of free radicals. In their topical form, these vitamins have recently been winging their way into skincare products. While vitamin-A derivatives (like Retinova) have been hailed as one of the biggest breakthroughs in cosmetic science, vitamin E, which is renowned for its nourishing effects, has long been a staple ingredient of anti-ageing products. More recently, however, vitamin C has created a wave of excitement among the cosmetic giants who have produced vitamin-C-enriched ranges which, by aiding the synthesis of collagen and defending against free radicals, claim to give skin a more youthful appearance. Cosmeceutical products like Cellex-C High Potency serum and C-Esta serum contain higher concentrates of vitamin C and are currently being used by some dermatologists to prepare their patients' skin for laser-resurfacing treatment. Other antioxidants gaining popularity include green tea, lycopene and extracts from grape-seed, pine bark, bilberry and the Chinese herb Schisandra fruit.

Retin-A

Proven to diminish wrinkles and reverse sun damage, Retin-A (also known as Tretinoin) is a vitamin-A-derivative skin drug which was originally prescribed as a treatment for acne, and which works by encouraging the peeling of the skin's outer layers. The anti-ageing benefits of Retin-A were discovered by chance when patients who were being treated for acne reported that the appearance of their wrinkles had improved. More recently, Retin-A derived preparations such as Retinova have been prescribed for the treatment of wrinkles, sun-damaged skin and uneven pigmentation.

Like most dermatologists, Dr Orentreich is a great fan of Retin-A, having seen its positive results time and time again. At present Retin-A preparations are only available on prescription from dermatologists or doctors. However, Retinol, a milder form, can now be found in over-the-counter cosmetics. Retin-A can cause skin redness, peeling and sun sensitivity, and all users are advised to wear a sunscreen.

Anti-wrinkle patches

First came the HRT (hormone-replacement therapy) patch; now cosmetic companies are spurning patches – wrinkle-zapping, transdermal pads, which are made of gauze impregnated with concentrated amounts of hydrating ingredients, such as vitamin C, petroleum jelly, wheatgerm oil and paraffin wax. When applied under the eyes, to the forehead or around the mouth, they plump up and soften the appearance of wrinkles. Results, however, are only temporary.

Skin peels

By sloughing off the top layers of skin, superficial skin peels can improve the look of such imperfections as acne scars, smooth out wrinkles and enhance the overall texture of the skin. One of the most widely used superficial skin-peeling agents is glycolic acid, an AHA which, when used in stronger concentrates, is employed for deeper chemical skin peels. Dr Orentreich, who uses another popular peeling agent, TCA (trichloroacetic acid), promotes the use of skin peels to improve the texture of the skin. Expect redness and mild peeling for a couple of days before a much softer, smoother skin is revealed. Milder glycolic-acid peels are also available in the form of peel facials at beauty salons. For deeper peels, see page 103.

The non-surgical face-lift

Electronic toning facials such as C.A.C.I. (computer-aided cosmetology instrument), Dibitron and O-Lys Light Therapy have been labelled face-lifts without surgery. With C.A.C.I., for example, a low-frequency microcurrent is delivered by means of twin probes (see picture right), allegedly toning the muscles and lifting the face. But can these machines really lift droopy eyelids, resculpture the face, diminish under-eye bags, erase lines and improve the skin's overall texture? I sent a fifty-one-year-old woman to act as a guinea pig and try the full C.A.C.I. course. Her response? 'Even though the jowls have not disappeared, C.A.C.I. did improve the texture of my skin and seemed to lift parts of my face.' In order to benefit from the non-surgical face-lift,

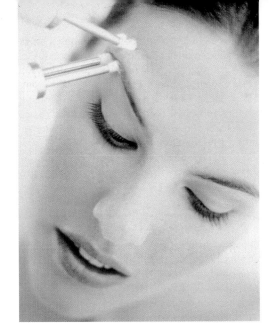

you need the full course of ten treatments and, as the results are only temporary, the downside is that you need regular maintenance sessions. While a non-surgical face-lift can make you look younger, it cannot help those areas that include loose skin or fat, such as jowls and double chins.

Those low-maintenance beauties who don't have the time for lengthy salon visits can purchase muscle-stimulating machines to use at home. These are either hand-held machines or, like Clio, ones that involve you sticking little pads onto your face and attaching them to wires. Those who flinch at the idea of being plugged in and switched on may prefer a natural, non-surgical face-lift, such as the Rejuvenessance technique. By using a gentle, finger-tip massage on specific parts of the face, the connective tissue is softened, which is said to help the skin regain its elasticity, restore mobility to the face, improve muscle tone and disperse toxins. This doesn't, however, have the same lifting effect as salon toners or facial exercises. Another non-electronic non-surgical face-lift is the Exoderm in which a phenol-based peel is applied to the face before the face is bandaged. Probably one of the best and cheapest non-surgical face-lifts is a facial workout (see page 106).

COSMETOLOGY

If you want to take your anti-ageing mission a step further than just using a facial serum, there is now an increasing number of minor cosmetic procedures which can help you to eradicate wrinkles and blemishes.

Whether you've got wrinkles or birthmarks, or simply want pouting lips and baby-smooth skin, there is now a whole host of state-of-the-art procedures, including dermal fillers, facial implants and various methods of skin resurfacing available. These procedures are not as invasive, nor do they carry the same level of risk and discomfort or the lengthy recovery time, as the more complex cosmetic surgery (see page 138). Nonetheless, they must all be carried out by a reputable dermatologist or plastic surgeon, otherwise you could run the risk of incurring skin sensitivity, allergic reactions, infection, burns, uneven pigmentation or even, in the worst-case scenario, facial disfigurement. Professor Nicholas Lowe, consultant dermatologist and clinical professor at the University of California at Los Angeles, is one of the world's leading dermatologists; he gives his advice throughout.

COSMETIC PROCEDURES

Dermal fillers
Dermal fillers treat lower facial lines and pitted acne scars and are also used for reshaping lips and plumping up hollow cheeks. Silicone was the first substance used but, as Professor Lowe explains: 'Due to risk of hardening, ulceration and an impossibility to remove, its use as a filler has become extremely limited.' Silicone was superseded by purified bovine collagen. 'Collagen has continued to be a mainstay dermal filler,' says Professor Lowe, 'although the results are only temporary, lasting between six and eighteen months, depending on the age and skin condition of the individual.' Because collagen carries a three per cent risk of inducing an allergy, dermatologists ought to perform a double patch test before administering it.

Other temporary fillers include Hylaform gel – a non-allergenic, synthetic substance that has both similar uses and results to collagen – and autologous lipotransfer, in which the patient's own fat is taken by means of painless liposuction from the stomach, hips, thighs, neck or lower face. 'With autologous fat fillers, we harvest the fat then, using microcanulas syringes, redeposit some of it into the face to fill in lines and hollow areas. The rest of the fat is frozen for future sessions,' explains Professor Lowe. He continues: 'As the process usually requires four to six injections given over several months, it's a lengthy procedure, but the benefits are long term, with sixty per cent of the fat remaining.'

Facial implants
The first facial-implant filler was Gore-Tex. 'We implant this biologically compatible membrane by threading it under the skin,' explains Professor Lowe. The most exciting and most recent implant is Softform. Developed by plastic surgeons at UCSF, this synthetic implant, which is made of expanded polytetrafluoroethylene, is a permanent solution. 'Softform is shaped into hollow tubes that feel natural when implanted,' says Professor Lowe. 'It also has the enormous advantage of being permanent yet, unlike Gore-Tex, dermis does not grow across the implant, so

it can easily be removed! The best sites for facial implants include the lips, the naso-labial folds, forehead furrows, marionette lines and crease lines on the chin. Any swelling and bruising, along with small sutures – stitches around the area where the Softform has been implanted – usually disappear within five days.

Botox

The bacteria toxin botulinum, most widely known as botox, has been used medically for years to treat stroke patients and people with eye twitches and squints. In the past few years, however, it has also become a fashionable line reducer, which is used to treat facial lines caused by the action of muscles. 'We inject a tiny amount of botox into the glabellar furrow [the crease between the eyebrows], which relaxes and immobilises the muscle, thus smoothing out lines and preventing further frowning,' says Professor Lowe. The process needs to be repeated three times within the first year, and then as often as necessary. Botox is also successful for smoothing out crow's-feet.

Liposculpture for the face

Liposculpture is a form of liposuction, which is used to remove the fatty deposits that are often to blame for jowls and double chins. 'Having applied local anaesthesia to the face, we extract the fat using a fine syringe', says Professor Lowe, who goes on to explain how shortly afterwards the skin tightens back. Patients must expect mild bruising and minor discomfort.

Skin rejuvenation

In the battle against lines and wrinkles, resurfacing areas of the face to reveal new, baby-soft skin has become extremely popular. 'Resurfacing gives you a new epidermis [top layer of skin],' explains Professor Lowe. Don't think that skin resurfacing is as simple as popping into the beauty salon for a facial, however: because the top layer of skin is literally burnt or peeled off, it can cause varying degrees of discomfort. Most physicians tend either to sedate their patients lightly, or to inject them with a local anaesthetic first. In some cases, when the entire face is treated, a general anaesthetic may be advised. The recovery time following skin resurfacing takes at least a week, during which patients must initially expect a sore, red face. After dermabrasion, laser resurfacing or a deep peel, a crust usually forms.

Chemical peels use peeling agents, such as trichloroacetic acid, glycolic acid, phenol or Jessner's solution, to improve moderate acne scars and reduce lines and wrinkles. 'The deeper peel is much more severe and involves the use of higher-strength peeling agents. We therefore give patients local anaesthesia and/or sedation,' says Professor Lowe. The drawbacks associated with deep chemical peels are that they do not penetrate as deep as the laser, and that all patients must wear a sunscreen after surgery, as there is a risk of skin discoloration.

A more drastic, and rather scary-sounding, resurfacing process is dermabrasion, a method in which skin is removed by rotating wire brushes. As this carries a risk of infection and involves a general anaesthetic, there is less demand for this procedure nowadays.

Laser rejuvenation has now eclipsed chemical peels and dermabrasion as the favourite procedure. 'The new lasers, such as the Ultrapulse CO_2 and the Erbium-Yag, provide excellent control and precision, which has made skin resurfacing faster healing and more effective,' says Professor Lowe, who is at the forefront of laser research. You could have your entire face resurfaced or else opt for resurfacing such specific zones as the under-eye area.

Moles, birthmarks and brown spots

The removal process for moles, birthmarks and brown spots (caused by sun exposure, ageing, pregnancy or the contraceptive pill) is quite simple, as the affliction can be lasered away with a Q-Switch Ruby laser. Professor Lowe warns, however, that moles should only be removed by a dermatologist or doctor because a beautician is not sufficiently qualified to be able to tell whether a mole is benign or not. 'I always carry out a biopsy to check if the mole is malignant. If this is the case, the mole must be surgically excised,' explains Professor Lowe.

FACE-SAVERS:
WAYS TO KNOCK YEARS OFF YOUR LOOKS

- **Protect your skin from the sun:** the sun is the number-one villain in ageing skin – exposure to it degenerates the skin's collagen and elastin fibres. A sunblock is your best defence.
- **Stop smoking:** smoking is the second most important cause of ageing. Because nicotine depletes the body's supply of vitamin C and deprives the cells of oxygen, the skin loses its elasticity and becomes thinner.
- **Fight stress:** stress accelerates ageing by slowing down the cell-renewal process.
- **Moderate your intake of tea, coffee, alcohol, sugar and junk food:** consuming excessive amounts will negatively affect the body's intake of essential vitamins and minerals.
- **Drink two litres of water a day:** if your body is thirsty it will rob the skin's cells of moisture, leaving the skin vulnerable to dehydration.
- **Age-proof your face:** invest in a good face cream that nourishes and protects your skin from the ravages of the environment.
- **Drink freshly-prepared vegetable juice:** it is packed with nutrients and is one of the best methods for improving your skin's health.
- **Fight line-forming free radicals:** pollution, drugs, smoking, radiation and sunlight exacerbate these cell-destroying molecules. To mop up excess numbers of free radicals, increase your intake of antioxidants.
- **Lubricate your skin from within:** do not cut fat out of your diet completely or you will find that your skin ages more rapidly. Introduce essential fatty acids (EFAs) into your diet by dressing salads with EFA rich oils (see page 178).
- **Exercise:** it increases the rate of cell production, oxygenates cells, tones the muscles and keeps skin looking younger.

- **Massage your face with cleanser:** to improve your skin tone, eliminate the build-up of toxins, relax tense muscles, boost blood circulation and promote cell renewal.
- **Exfoliate your skin:** as we get older the skin-renewal process slows down, so we need to slough off dead cells in order to encourage cell production and improve the skin's texture.
- **Breathe deeply:** this is essential for oxygenating cells. Also, get plenty of fresh air.
- **Step up your nutritional intake:** strengthen your skin's defences by eating a healthy, balanced diet, including plenty of raw, fresh fruit and vegetables. You could also include anti-ageing supplements in your diet. Some of the supplements available include antioxidants: vitamin A, C and E, grape-seed and pine bark extracts; GLA supplements: evening-primrose or borage oil; as well as cod liver oil, wheatgrass, selenium, spectrumzyme and full-spectrum amino acids.
- **Keep your environment healthy:** in stuffy, centrally-heated and air-conditioned offices a humidifier – or even just a bowl of water – will help prevent your skin from becoming dehydrated. Keep your home well ventilated.
- **Prevent sleep lines by sleeping on your back:** if you can't sleep in this position, apply a dab of Vaseline Petroleum Jelly to areas that are vulnerable, such as your neck and décolletage.
- **Control your facial expressions:** try to refrain from frowning or squinting habitually.
- **Smile:** you'll look years younger. (Marlene Dietrich was once overheard telling a young, up-and-coming actress: 'When you are young, never smile – it causes wrinkles. But when you are old, smile all the time – it hides them.')

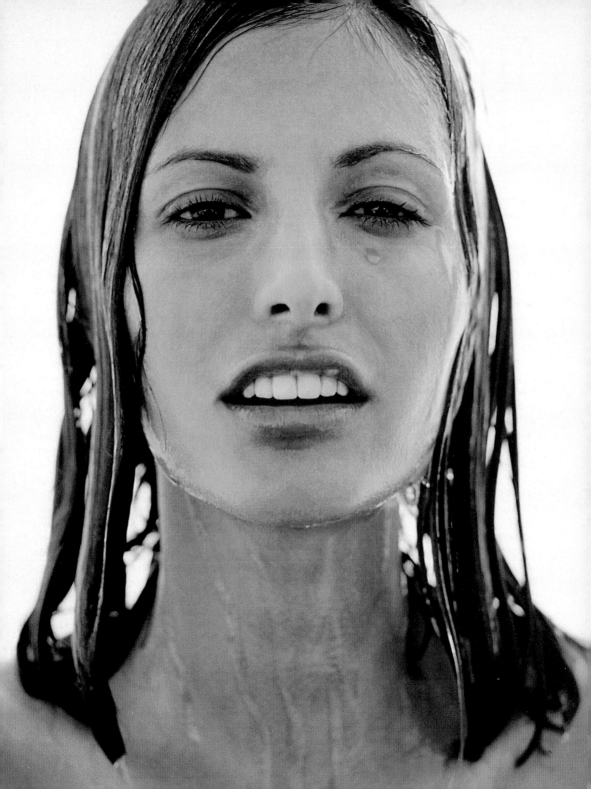

THE FACIAL WORKOUT

Like the idea of chiselled cheekbones, pouty lips and taut skin,
with no sags, bags or jowls? Facial fitness is the key.

Ever since I interviewed the pioneer of facial exercises, Eva Fraser, I have been pulling ferociously funny faces in front of the mirror. Within a matter of weeks of starting, there was a noticeable improvement in both my muscle tone and complexion, and I definitely had higher cheekbones. However, Eva told me that it would take up to six months to see the real results of moulding my facial contours and lifting my face in this way. There's no doubt that you need to be dedicated – these exercises certainly aren't for the low-maintenance beauty. But take one look at Eva (see picture below), who at seventy has razor-sharp cheekbones and not a wrinkle, under-eye bag or droopy bit of skin in sight, and you'll realise that just a few

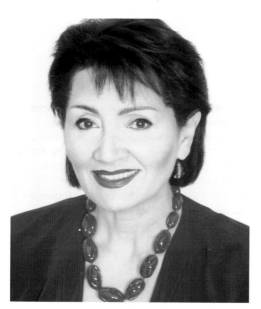

minutes' workout a day pays dividends. The beauty of facial exercises is you can do them anywhere: you don't have to visit a salon and they are also a cost-free way of looking good.

Facial aerobics make sense: anyone who exercises regularly will know that it is possible to improve your muscle tone and even resculpture your physique. 'The facial muscles are just like the body's,' explains Eva, 'yet most of us haven't used them since we lay screaming in our cots.' Her method uses a series of small, precise movements which work on shortening fourteen facial muscles.

Some sceptics believe that facial exercises can potentially cause lines created by habitual muscular overuse, but as Eva points out: 'You often smile or frown a hundred times a day yet, when you are exercising your face, you only repeat a facial expression a few times'. Top plastic surgeon Basim Matti refers his patients to Eva and comments: 'I admire the method and, although there is no science to back it up, it certainly seems to improve muscle tone.'

Prevention is always better than cure, so the younger you start exercising your face the better. Even so, my mother didn't discover facial exercises until she was fifty and looks better now than she did a decade ago. Exercising fights against gravitational pull, keeping the facial muscles taut and preventing the drooping that causes bags and sags. As Eva points out, however, once the skin has become so slack that it has separated from the connective tissue, there is little that you can do to improve it. And, if the sagging is caused by fatty deposits in areas like jowls or under the chin, facial exercises cannot help that either.

THREE OF EVA FRASER'S BEST FACIAL EXERCISES

Here is a taster of three of Eva's exercises. To benefit fully from her facial exercises, follow Eva's full workout which is demonstrated in *Facial Fitness* (Facial Fitness Centre Ltd., 1998) a video, audio and book package.

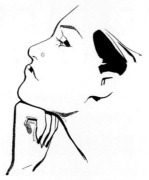

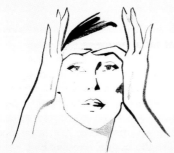

1 The upper-eyelid exercise: to lift the eye area

With age, the upper eye muscles become weak, allowing excess skin to droop over the eyes. This simple exercise puts the springiness back into the eye area by smoothing out folds in the upper eyelids, preventing the outer corners from sagging and keeping the eyebrows up.

1 Look into a mirror throughout the exercise.
2 Curve your index finger along your brow line, just under your eyebrow. Now gently push your finger up and hold it against your brow bone.
3 Close eyes, stretching upper eyelids in a downward direction in five small steps.
4 Hold the position for a count of six.
5 Release the tension slowly in three counts. Repeat twice.

2 The 'turkey-neck' eliminator: for a firm neck and jaw line

Double chins, a slack jaw line and loose, turkey-like skin on the neck can look unattractive and incredibly ageing. The muscle which runs under the chin slackens over the years, but by doing this exercise once a day, you can train it to become taut again or, better still, prevent it from slackening in the first place.

1 Look into a mirror throughout the exercise.
2 Raise your chin up and, at the same time, draw the centre of your bottom lip up over your top lip. (Do not smile by lifting up the corners of your mouth – remember that you are bringing up the centre of your bottom lip.)
3 Holding this position, press the tip of your tongue against the outside of lower teeth.
4 Now thrust your chin and tongue forward as if you were taking off in Concorde.
5 Hold the position for a count of six, then slowly release it. Repeat twice.

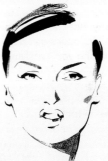

3 Kissing the mirror: for full lips and superb cheekbones

This simple little exercise works wonders, shaping your lower cheeks, helping to tighten your jowls and making your lips look fuller.

1 Look into a mirror throughout the exercise.
2 Place the flat parts of your index fingers on the corners of your mouth, then slide them back for an inch on each side and hold the position firmly.
3 Bring your lips forward into a pout.
4 Make an exaggerated kissing gesture as though you were kissing the mirror (take care not to pucker your top lip). Repeat ten times.

FACIALS

WHAT ARE THE BENEFITS?

The Aveda facial has been described as better than sex: as you're being pampered into an heavenly state your skin is anointed with all sorts of potions and lotions, is smothered in masks, stimulated, massaged, exfoliated and relaxed. Although some people still view facials as a one-off treat or a quick fix for parched or problem skin, regular facials are a must if you want to maintain a good complexion. If I had the time and money I would love one a week but, according to beauty therapists, one a month is perfectly adequate.

Nothing quite beats the relaxed and pampered feeling you get from having a salon facial, but the true benefits of going to a salon come from firstly, the therapist's experience, and secondly, the salon's equipment and the professional products that are used. However, by using just a few specialised products, or even home-made recipes (see page 164), you can perform your own facial at home.

CHOOSING A FACIAL

With their costs ranging from £15 to £100, facial treatments do not come cheap, so make sure that you pick a good facial, like one of the leading salon facials offered by such cosmetic companies as Decleor, Guinot, Clarins, Elemis, Thalgo, E'spa, Gatineau, Dermalogica, Aveda, Elizabeth Arden, WU! and Pier Auge.

I once made the mistake of going off the beaten beauty track only to experience a facial nightmare. The beautician stuck on a steamer, which proceeded to gurgle and spit boiling water at me. She then left me for twenty minutes, before returning to massage my face clumsily, a procedure which, to make matters worse, was interrupted every time the phone rang. Having slapped on a mask, she then disappeared. Instead of leaving you alone while your mask sets, many therapists now continue pampering you throughout: at Aveda, for example, your hands and feet are massaged, while E'spa's therapists gently stimulate your scalp.

TYPES OF FACIALS

There are dozens of variations on the facial, from the basic, deep-cleansing version to the holistic facial that treats the face, neck, back and scalp. While some salon treatments involve the use of electrical equipment, others prefer to take a hands-on approach or else combine the two procedures to create the perfect New Age facial. The products that are smoothed over the face also differ – generally they are either made from plant extracts, aromatherapy- or marine-based products. When choosing a facial, remember to take your skin type into consideration: a hydrating treatment could aggravate oily, spotty skin, whereas a deep-cleansing facial may be exactly what your skin is crying out for.

Before you plunder the yellow pages or your beauty address book, let me tell you about the main facial procedures available. A popular deep-cleansing facial is Guinot's Catheodermie, in which a galvanic, high-frequency current is used to purify the skin and help it absorb treatment creams. Another favourite procedure is the vacuum facial, which cleanses the pores by sucking blackheads into a tube. With the holistic approach now at the forefront of health and beauty philosophies, it's not surprising that the holistic facial has become a firm favourite among facialphiles. Taking the concept of the facial further, the beautician treats not only your face, but also massages your scalp, shoulders, neck and back. Shiatsu and French massage are two of the massage techniques used in facials.

Most facials incorporate some form of exfoliation, but you can take this a step further by having a salon facial peel, in which the overall texture of the skin is improved by removing layers of skin with low-level solutions of glycolic or another AHA acid. AHA peels are not the only salon skin rejuivinators; another method blasts skin with fine crystals, while ultra sound micro-vibrations administered via a metal instrument is a less aggressive way of sloughing off dead skin. Anti-ageing electronic and light-therapy facials, which tone and firm the face and give the skin a more youthful appearance, are becoming increasingly in demand (see page 101), while oxygen facials, in which pure oxygen is delivered from a tank in blasts to the skin to help reactivate skin cells, are also popular.

THE HOME FACIAL

You will need: a face cloth (preferably made of muslin), a cleanser, toner and moisturiser, a facial exfoliator, face mask, massage oil and a water-based misting product (see page 164 to make your own DIY preparations).

- **Cleanse:** remove all traces of stale make-up and grime by cleansing your face thoroughly. Run your face cloth under warm water, wring it out and then cover your face with it for a few seconds. Repeat this procedure three times to soften your skin. Alternatively, you could steam your face by adding a few herbs and drops of essential oils to boiling water, or by using a ready-prepared product, such as Dr Hauschka's Steam Bath Concentrate. Steam for about five minutes. (Do not steam your face if you are susceptible to thread veins.)
- **Exfoliate:** spend a few minutes massaging a gentle facial scrub into your face to remove dead skin cells. (For a DIY exfoliant see page 164.)
- **Facial massage:** using a facial oil, like E'spa's Balancing Facial Oil, Decleor's Aromessence Visage Neroli Oil or a vegetable oil, such as wheatgerm, olive or avocado, massage the whole of your face using small, circular movements for ten minutes.
- **Mask:** use a mask that suits your skin's needs. A hydrating mask, for example, will replace lost moisture, whereas if you want a deep cleanse, a deep-penetrating mask will help to lift out any impurities and will leave your skin scrupulously clean. (Try one of the DIY masks on page 164.)
- **Eye pads:** leave your face mask on for fifteen to twenty minutes and, in the meantime, treat your under-eye area by either applying a hydrating eye mask, refreshing eye pads, cucumber slices or cold tea bags.
- **Tone and moisturise:** rinse off all traces of the mask and spritz your face with a soothing, water-based mist, such as E'spa's Herbal Spa Fresh, Decleor's Floral Moisturising Spray or Vichy's Eau Thermale, before smothering on a light layer of moisturiser.

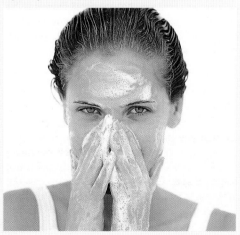

EYECARE

Eyes are the windows of your soul;
treat them well and they will sparkle.

GENERAL EYECARE TIPS

- The thinnest, most delicate skin of all lies around the eye area, so eye products and make-up should be applied with the utmost care and the lightest possible touch.
- Apply an eye cream or gel that has been specially formulated for the eye area both morning and night. (A facial moisturiser is too heavy for this delicate area and will clog the pores causing whiteheads and puffiness.)
- When applying eye cream or gel, gently tap a tiny dot of the preparation just inside the socket bone with your fourth finger. This is as close as you need to get; your body heat will encourage the cream to migrate towards the eye.
- Never apply eye cream or gel to your eyelids: the product could seep into your eyes and cause irritation.
- Remove your eye make-up with a specially formulated eye make-up remover, not your regular cleanser. Using a dampened piece of cotton wool, smooth it gently over your eyes. Contact lense wearers should remove lenses before taking off eye make-up.
- When applying concealer or eyeshadow, take care not to drag the skin. Brushes are ideal as they make blending easier.
- To avoid irritation, wash brushes, sponges and other make-up applicators regularly, and never share eye make-up.
- Unless it's for the odd special occasion, as a general rule you should not apply eyeliner to the inside rims of eyes, as it can cause infection and irritate the eyes.
- Prevent eye strain by getting your eyes tested every three to five years.

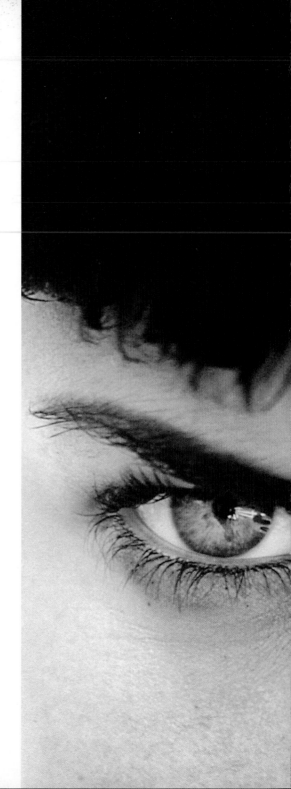

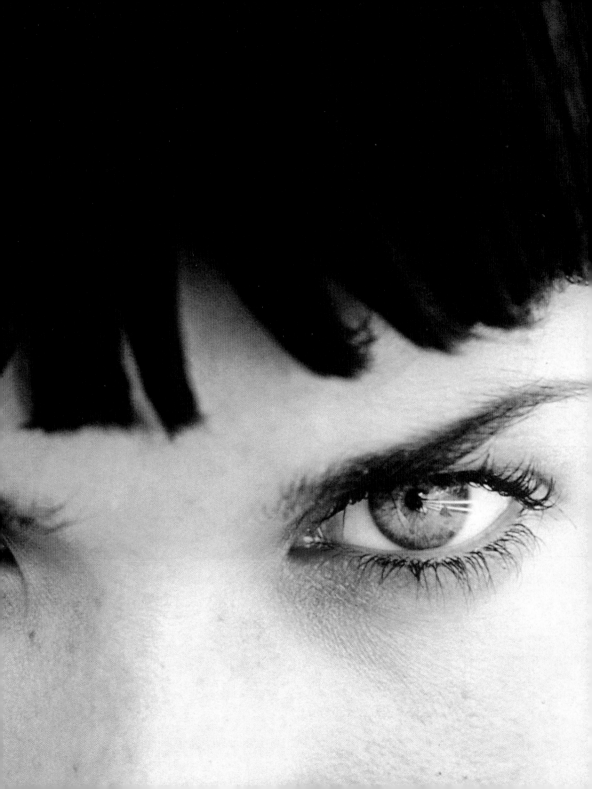

BRIGHTEN UP YOUR EYES

Your eyes reflect the state of your health and your lifestyle. Such varied factors as a poor diet, illness, hay fever, allergies, lack of sleep and staring at the computer screen, take their toll on the whole optical area, resulting in yellowish eye whites, bloodshot eyes and other problems, like redness and puffiness both above and below the eyes.

Solutions

• Bathe your eyes in an eye solution for thirty seconds once daily until they return to normal. Try Dr Hauschka's Eye Freshener Concentrate, Optrex's Eye Bath or make up your own saline solution by dissolving half a teaspoon of salt into 300ml of mineral water.

• To brighten your eye whites instantly, use whitening drops, such as D.R. Harris', Visine's or Optrex's – these contain a vascoconstrictor to help shrink red capillaries. Avoid using too often, however, as overuse can cause the capillaries to dilate permanently.

• Don't sit too close to computer screens; they are notorious for straining eyes.

• Read in a good light to prevent eye strain.

• Try the following eye exercise: look to the right, then the left; now look up and down. Repeat this procedure five times.

• Ensure that you always remove every scrap of eye make-up before you go to bed or you could wake up with sore, red eyes.

• Rest your eyes using the 'palming' technique: close your eyes and cup the palms of your hands over your eyes for at least one minute.

• Soothe your eyes by applying cotton-wool pads that have been soaked in witch hazel or milk. Leave on for ten minutes.

• If your eyes become sensitive or itchy, check that you are not allergic to any eyecare products, such as eye creams, gels, eye make-up remover, contact lense solution or eye make-up. If you suspect that one of them is causing irritation, you should be able to determine the trigger irritant by means of a process of elimination, that is, by not wearing one of your regular products for at least a couple of days.

BANISH PUFFINESS

Under-eye puffiness can be triggered by a number of factors, including water retention, allergies, colds, constipation, sleep deprivation, the overuse of eye products and even too much sleep. A damp environment can also exacerbate the problem (the day that I moved out of a damp basement flat my under-eye bags diminished). However, if under-eye bags or puffiness seem to be with you permanently, pockets of fat or slack muscles could be the culprits; short of surgery, there is little that you can do to solve this problem.

Solutions

• Gentle massage around the eye area will help to promote fluid drainage, oxygenate cells and alleviate puffiness. Lightly tap around the eye socket and brow bone daily with your index finger, tapping twenty times on each spot.

• Use an eye gel or balm rather than cream in the mornings, such as Swisscare Pour Givenchy's Double Sequence Eye Contour Firming Balm, Erno Lazlo's pHelitone Firmly Eye Gel Mask, YSL's Smoothing Eye Contour Gel or Synergie's Eye Gel Bio-Contour.

• For an instant fix, lie down for ten minutes and cover eyes with a cold, refreshing eye mask, such as The Body Shop's Blue Gel Mask or Borghese's Eye Compresses. DIY alternatives include cucumber, raw potato slices or chilled tea bags.

• If you think that your puffiness could be due to water retention, cut down on salty, spicy and smoked foods and alcohol.

• Try sleeping either with an extra pillow or with the top of your bed raised a few inches – the elevation will encourage drainage.

• Drink at least two litres of water a day to help your body to eliminate any waste products and toxins that could be provoking the condition; this will also help to prevent water retention.

• Eye products, face creams or make-up could be triggering puffiness. Do not apply products too close to eyes and try switching brands.

• Permenant under-eye puffiness caused by pockets of fat can be effectively removed by lower-eye surgery (see page 139).

COMBAT DARK SHADOWS

If you look like you've been in the ring with Mike Tyson and wouldn't dare to leave home without wearing concealer, then you are probably the victim of under-eye shadows. For some people this is an inherited condition which is caused by darker pigmentation in the eye area. Dark circles are yet another sign of the ravages of age, too: as you grow older, the skin around the eyes becomes thinner, thus making the underlying blood vessels and veins more apparent. If you have fair or transparent skin, superficial veins are also more noticeable. But remember that dark circles can simply be a temporary occurrence: sinusitis, a sluggish liver, lack of sleep, illness, allergies and poor waste elimination are some of the key short-term factors that can prohibit the correct functioning of the skin's tiny blood vessels, and result in a darkening of the area.

Solutions

• If your dark shadows are temporary, try to establish and then tackle the cause of problem. (You could even have a general health check in order to identify and consequently address any underlying health problems that you may have.)

• Apply an eye cream that has a lightening effect, such as Avon's Lighten Up Under-eye Cream, Estée Lauder's Uncircle Eye Treatment, Prescriptives Uplift or Laura Mercier's Secret Camoflage.

• Conceal dark circles with a light-reflective foundation or concealer, such as YSL's Touche Éclat or Colourings' Lightening Touch.

• Go to bed half an hour earlier than usual.

• If your dark circles are the result of sinus problems, try raising the top of your bed by a few inches. Inhaling euculyptus oil can also help decongest sinuses.

• Cold compresses – cucumber slices, chilled tea bags or a cooling eye mask straight from the fridge – will temporarily shrink blood vessels and help lighten up the under-eye area.

• Include plenty of fibrous foods in your diet, as constipation can lead to dark circles.

• The pigmentation that causes dark circles can effectively be reduced with a laser.

CONTROL LINES, CROW'S-FEET AND CREPINESS

Perhaps you think yourself lucky enough to have escaped puffiness and dark circles around your eyes, but unless you refrain from smiling for the rest of your life, it is impossible to avoid accumulating laughter lines around the eye, which often form in the shape of crow's-feet. Under-eye lines are also the result of exposure to the sun, squinting and even the position in which you sleep.

The skin surrounding the eye is particularly fragile, being thinner and having fewer glands than the rest of the face. Because it is also more prone to dryness, lines, wrinkles and crepiness, as the membranes get weaker and the skin loses its elasticity, the eye zone is also the first to show signs of ageing. But, by taking good care of this area and protecting it from the harsh effects of the elements, you can keep lines, crow's-feet and crepiness at bay.

Solutions

• Apply a good eye cream both morning and night. Try Shiseido's Vital Perfection Daily Eye Primer, Lancaster's Oxygen Supply for Eyes, Nivea Visage's Anti Wrinkle Eyezone Q10 Repair Cream or L'Oréal's Plenitude Contour Regard Eye Cream.

• Give your under-eye skin an extra boost by applying a treatment prior to your eye cream. Guerlain's Issima Eye Serum, Elizabeth Arden's Ceramides Eye Capsules and Cellex-C Eye Contour Gel are three good treatments.

• Once a week, treat your eyes to a nourishing eye mask, such as Kanebo's Eye Mask Elixir or Clarins' Skin Smoothing Eye Mask. Plump up under-eye skin and temporarily reduce lines by means of anti-wrinkle patches (see page 101).

• Avoid sleep lines and creases by sleeping on your back.

• Crow's-feet can be improved with laser resurfacing (see page 103).

• Wear sunglasses, even on a sunny winter's day, to protect your eye area from the sun's rays and prevent the formation of sun- and squinting-induced lines and crow's-feet.

THE HOLLYWOOD SMILE

A dazzling display of pearly white teeth will do wonders for your image, not to mention your self-confidence. But if the tooth fairy left you with a set of yellow, stained or crooked teeth, don't worry: nowadays you can design your own Hollywood smile.

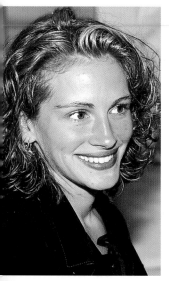

SMILE MAKE-OVERS

It is now possible to buy a designer smile: in just the same way as you may show your hairdresser a picture of a hairstyle you want, according to dentist to the stars Dr Marc Lowenberg, from the Lowenberg and Lituchy Dental Office in New York, you can replicate a model or celebrity's smile by changing the size, position, length and colour of your teeth using such techniques as veneering and reshaping.

'To achieve a broad, Julia Roberts'-like smile – where practically every tooth in the mouth is on show – we widen arches and veneer the outsides of the teeth,' says Dr Lowenberg. 'Another desired celebrity smile is Claudia Schiffer's. Her two front teeth are longer, which is in itself sexy. This also has the effect of making her top lip curl up, giving her a sultry pout. If someone wants a sexy smile, we might lengthen the two front teeth with veneers or reshape the adjacent teeth.'

The anti-ageing smile

Rejuvenating your smile can knock years off your age, but you don't need a set of false teeth in order to do this. According to Dr Lowenberg, the ageing process causes our smile to change: 'As muscle tone slackens, the upper lip droops and covers the top teeth, while the lower lip droops to reveal bottom teeth. Over the years, teeth also wear down, becoming shorter and darker. We therefore rebuild using veneers, and reshape the teeth to the size they were when the patient was twenty. The veneers also have the added value of supporting sagging muscle.'

COSMETIC PROCEDURES

● **Teeth whitening:** discoloration occurs deep within the tooth's structure and cannot be simply scrubbed off with whitening toothpaste, although this is effective in removing stains. By having your teeth professionally bleached you can glisten like the Colgate girl. The procedure lasts for a good couple of years and, according to Dr Lowenberg – who even bleaches his children's teeth – won't damage your teeth. DIY bleaching kits are available to buy but, as Dr Lowenberg points out: 'The level of bleach is low, and you will not get the same effect as having your teeth whitened by your dentist.'

● **Aesthetic contouring:** 'Dentists can reshape teeth by filing. Shaping is also good for softening pointed eye-teeth or squaring teeth to make them look more dynamic,' says Dr Lowenberg.

● **Straightening and realigning:** adjusting the alignment of the teeth with braces is not only used for straightening teeth, but can also correct and realign the jaw area. It's a lengthy process – taking from six months to two years – but wearers don't have to worry about being nicknamed 'metal-mouth': braces are far more discreet these days – some match tooth colour, while others are attached to the back of the teeth.

- **Gum trimming:** dentists can either contour the gums to reveal longer teeth or can level up an uneven gum line.
- **Veneers:** 'Veneers are the best thing that ever happened in cosmetic dentistry,' says Dr Lowenberg. 'We use them to correct a myriad of problems, including altering the shape of a tooth, straightening crooked or crossed teeth, closing up gaps, lengthening or covering a discoloured tooth.' Rather like a false nail, a porcelain veneer is bonded to the underlying tooth, which is filed down by only half a millimetre. Although veneers are thinner than crowns, according to Dr Lowenberg, they still have a long life span.
- **Implants:** these false, screw-in teeth are made from titanium and screwed into a metal device which has been implanted into the bone. If the bone is solid, the success rate is high but, then again, so is the price!
- **Crowns:** although crowns are still used to cover badly broken teeth or to replace old ones, they have generally given way to veneers. The crowning procedure means that more of the tooth is filed down, leaving only a peg, which is then covered with a cap. Old crowns are replaced either if the gum has receded or if the natural teeth have darkened. Modern crowns are made from pure porcelain and are therefore far more natural-looking than their metal predecessors.
- **Bonding:** tooth-coloured substance is used either for filling in gaps or bonding onto a tooth.

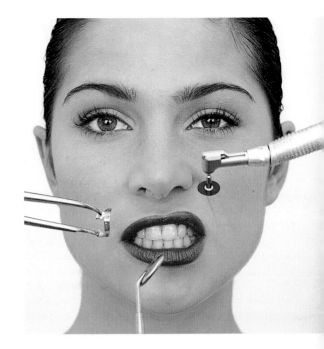

- **Fillings:** most dentists are now using white fillings as alternatives to amalgam-metal fillings. White fillings made from composite resin are the most common but, as Dr Lowenberg points out, if you want a perfect colour match you may want to splash out on porcelain alternatives.
- **Bridges:** to fill in gaps, artificial porcelain teeth are attached to a metal bridge and fitted between two crowned teeth.

TEN STEPS TOWARDS GAINING A DAZZLING SMILE

1 Floss your teeth daily with dental floss or Y-shaped, plastic-framed flossers.

2 Clean your teeth thoroughly two or three times daily for at least two minutes, using a fluoride toothpaste.

3 Consider investing in an electric toothbrush: it will clean your teeth more thoroughly.

4 Have any amalgam-metal fillings replaced with white alternatives.

5 Visit your dentist every six months.

6 Have your teeth professionally cleaned regularly, a procedure which includes scaling (to remove plaque and stains) and polishing.

7 Avoid encouraging decay by cutting sugary foods and drinks out of your diet and always cleaning your teeth after eating fruit or drinking fruit juice.

8 Remove stains caused by nicotine, coffee and red wine with a whitening toothpaste.

9 Change your toothbrush every three months.

10 Use a mouthwash to keep your mouth bacteria-free.

HOW TO ACHIEVE A MODEL-PERFECT
COMPLEXION

Why is it that supermodels and celebrities don't seem to have a spot or wrinkle in sight? What is their secret? Here you can discover how you, too, can have an enviably flawless complexion.

Let's get something straight: models may have the benefit of soft camera lenses and flattering lighting, not to mention having their photographs retouched with an airbrush or computer but, when looking at their pictures, don't be deceived into thinking that their flawless complexions are only the result of clever manipulation. Models are, by no means, immune to the occasional spot, but they certainly have it sussed when it comes to skincare, paying zealous attention to their skincare routines and arming themselves against all the major skin offenders – the sun, pollution, smoking, stress and alcohol.

A great-looking complexion is determined by skin that is firm, plump, smooth and has a radiant bloom. Think of a child's face: it is neither oily nor dry, just balanced. We all had such perfect skin once, before the skin-damaging culprits robbed us of it. However, top facialist Jo Malone, whose clients include Yasmin Le Bon, Gail Elliot and Lulu, insists that a healthy complexion is within everyone's reach with a little dedication and discipline.

If achieving a flawless complexion seems to elude you, start to optimise your skin's functioning by taking Jo's advice and sticking to a good routine. Cherish your skin by shielding your face from the sun, and counteracting the constant onslaught of dietary chemicals and pollution by combining wholesome nutrition with regular exercise and adequate sleep. Skin undoubtedly benefits from regular doses of tender loving care, but your lifestyle and how you look after yourself are equally important, too. If you smoke, are rarely seen without a drink in your hand, eat junk food and bombard your skin with ultraviolet rays, you may as well forget about having a beautiful complexion.

ASSESS YOUR SKIN

Unless you are one of the lucky few who has been blessed with perfectly balanced skin, it is unlikely that your skin will remain one type for long. Many factors can cause skin to change its type: in one month alone, for instance, it can flit from being ultra-dry, due to central heating, to being oily during menstruation. Throw in a skiing trip or beach holiday and it could be constantly yo-yoing between types; and whichever product works one week may be ineffective the next.

Leading skincare consultant Eve Lom believes that skin rarely falls into one general type. She therefore stresses that you should constantly review your skin's condition and be your own therapist: 'You know your skin better than anyone else, so you should be able to assess it.' Having assessed your skin, you need to treat it accordingly. If your moisturiser is too

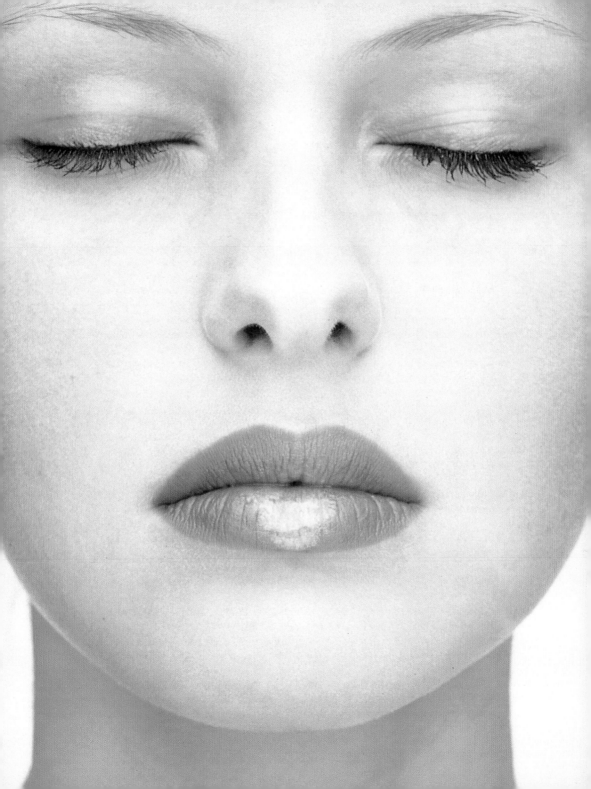

heavy, for example, dilute it by adding a little water to your hands before application. While your foaming facial wash is no doubt ideal for summer, during the winter months you might want to use a cleanser with a richer consistency to protect your skin against the drying effects of cold weather. Or it may be that your skin has become so sensitive to hi-tech products that it needs something more soothing.

HOW TO USE PRODUCTS

You may have dipped into your savings for a pot of prized cleanser or face cream, but if you slap it on willy-nilly you could both be doing your skin more harm than good and, what's more, undermining the product's performance. Skin is a remarkable organ which, when left to its own devices, will moisturise and cleanse itself. With cosmetic companies selling extra products for upteen procedures, however, it's easy to succumb to their lure. But overzealous cleansing and using copious amounts of moisturisers, masks and serums will upset the skin's delicate balance and do more harm than good.

After cleansing, the best way in which to ensure that all the residue is removed is to rinse your face with water; wiping your skin with a toner will make doubly sure of this. Rather than hurriedly applying your face cream, Jo suggests that after toning you should leave your face alone for one minute before moisturising it: 'This breather gives the skin time to get ready to accept the moisturiser.' Moisturising is where most people go wrong: if they are overgenerous, for example, moisturiser can inhibit the skin's natural functioning, leaving it puffy, congested and undermining its capacity to remain firm. One question that Jo is often asked is how much moisturiser to use and where to use it? 'My advice is, if after pulling a funny face your skin feels taut, you have not used enough. Before you apply any serum or moisturiser your face should be slightly warmed or the product will just sit on the skin and not be absorbed. Massage the moisturiser into your skin, not forgetting your lips and neck, but ensure that you keep it well away from your eye area.'

A TWICE-DAILY MASSAGE REGIME

Massage is both the basis of good skincare and, according to Jo, the key skin preserver. It improves the skin's tone and the efficiency of cleansing, activates its metabolism, stimulates blood circulation, encourages the oxygen supply to cells and, by breaking down pockets of fluid and fatty deposits, also helps to decongest the skin.

Jo, like many other facialists, believes that massage should be an essential part of everyone's daily skincare regime and has therefore devised a simple massage technique for her clients. For best results, Jo recommends using her own cleansing milk and repeating the regime morning and night. A couple of hints: never massage dry skin. And it's no good just tickling your face: for the massage to be effective you need to apply some pressure. If you are massaging your skin correctly, your face should have a healthy glow to it.

Step 1   Splash your face with water, before smoothing cleanser over your face and neck.

Step 2   Using two middle fingers, start massaging your face in upward, circular movements, sliding your fingers along your cheeks, across the forehead and around the nasal area, not forgetting the neck. Do this for between thirty and sixty seconds.

Step 3   Wipe away any remnants of cleanser, washing your face if you wish. Towel-dry your face and continue with your skincare regime.

Perfect skin – it's all in the mind

A final word about achieving a flawless complexion: we know that the mind and the skin are intrinsically linked and that mental stress can manifest itself in such skin conditions as acne and eczema. Eve Lom strongly believes that a positive attitude can benefit your skin: 'Accept your spot and it will go away; get paranoid about it and you'll end up with a whole crop of them.' Perhaps that explains why we always manage to get a spot in the most eye-drawing place precisely when we want to look our best for a hot date or important interview!

DECIPHERING THE JARGON

'Hypo-allergenic' and 'allergy tested', or terms to this effect, imply that the product has been tested for skin sensitivity. 'Fragrance-free' means exactly what it says, while 'dermatologically approved' or 'dermatologically tested' indicate that the product has been tested on human skin. 'Non-acnedemic' and 'non-comedogenic' – words found mainly on moisturisers and foundations – claim to keep your pores unclogged and therefore prevent spots. You may also have noticed the words 'pH balanced' on the packaging of some cleansers: the pH level refers your skin's acid mantle which, when balanced, should be at about 5.5.

'Has not been tested on animals', 'cruelty free' or 'tested on models not animals', are thankfully statements that we are seeing more and more of on beauty-products' packaging.

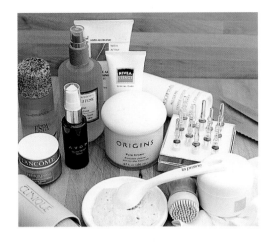

However, as the staple ingredients found in most cosmetics were tested on animals in the past, the wording you are most likely to find is: 'This product has not been tested on animals'.

SKINCARE DOS AND DON'TS

Do understand your skin's needs. Be guided by any changes in the condition of your skin and use the right products to treat it accordingly.

Do spend a minute or so massaging your cleanser into your face – among other things massage improves cleansing efficiency.

Do use a serum or special-treatment cream (once in a while, not continuously) if your skin is in extra need of nourishment.

Do exfoliate your skin regularly, using either a gentle facial exfoliant, face cloth or facial peel.

Do use a mask once a week.

Do leave skin naked – free of make-up or cream – for a few minutes each day to allow it to breathe.

Do carry out a patch test on every new product before using it in order to check that you aren't allergic to it: apply the product to the inside of your elbow for at least three days.

Do extend your cleansing, moisturising and exfoliating regime to your neck.

Do apply moisturiser and eye cream before putting on foundation.

Don't scrub your face with anything too harsh – hard exfoliant grains can scratch the skin.

Don't wash your face in very hot water or splash it with ice-cold water: these extremes in temperature can cause thread veins.

Don't leave water or toner on your face or it will dehydrate your skin – instead, tissue it off.

Don't continue using any skincare product if it is causing an adverse reaction, such as blotchiness, swelling or irritation, regardless of how much it cost, and whether or not its formulation is based on natural ingredients or claims to be 'hypo-allergenic'.

Don't swamp your skin with cream as this will undermine its natural functioning.

Don't use soap: it leaves a residue, dehydrates and disturbs the skin's pH balance.

Don't drag your skin when cleansing.

Don't keep switching products. As skin takes time to adjust, you'll benefit if you finish the pot.

Don't use alcohol-based toners or harsh, antibacterial washes, as these products will strip the skin of its natural oils.

SKINCARE REGIMES

Cleanse

The cornerstone of skincare is cleansing, so don't underestimate the importance of cleansing your skin thoroughly in order to remove grime, stale make-up and dead skin cells. When cleansing, spend an extra minute massaging the product into your face to boost your skin's blood circulation and aid decongestion. Many facialists, like Eve Lom and Jo Malone, stress the importance of removing all traces of cleanser and encourage the use of a brush or face cloth when doing this, thereby adding an exfoliating dimension to the cleansing process. If you want to use a face cloth, Eve suggests one made of muslin, which is inexpensive and can be bought either from haberdashery stores or from chemists (in 'nappy' form, which can be chopped into squares).

Cleansers now come in many different versions, from a traditional cleansing lotion to a state-of-the-art foaming facial wash. Finding the right cleanser that both suits your skin and lifestyle is vital, or you could end up doing more harm than good. Facial washes (in both gel and creamy formulations) and cleansing bars are great if you prefer to wash rather than wipe, but are more suitable for morning use or for make-up-free skin. Always rinse thoroughly, splashing your face several times. If you wear make-up, you are better off using a wipe-off, oil-based lotion.

All those who are still using soap (not cleansing bars, which are soap-free) are committing a serious beauty crime, so throw it away and consider using one of the many different types of cleansers available, such as Jo Malone's Cleansing Milk and Complexion Brush, Eve Lom's Cleansing Cream, Origins' Pure Rinse Cream, Clinique's Facial Soap, Neutrogena's Cleansing Bar, Guinot's Refreshing Cleansing Milk and Shu Uemura's Cleansing Beauty Oil Fresher.

Exfoliate

Although it didn't appear in beauty books a decade ago, the word 'exfoliation' has become an integral part of our skincare vocabulary. Skin renews itself naturally every twenty-one days or so anyway (although such factors as the environment and ageing can slow this process down). But the reason why we've become obsessed with exfoliating is because it performs a multitude of actions: sloughing away dead cells, smoothing the skin, allowing it to breathe, improving its tone and even speeding up the rate of cell turnover. An exfoliated face is also more receptive to creams and treatments.

Like all good things, however, moderation is advisable when exfoliating. And, you don't necessarily need to use a gritty facial scrub: a peel or even a rub with a rough towel or face cloth works just as effectively. The aim is to remove any dead cells from the skin's surface without disturbing the healthy cells beneath; overdo it, and you'll be buffing away those skin cells that are not yet ready to go. The current skincare darlings, AHAs, BHAs and enzymes, are known for their exfoliating action and are found in many exfoliant preparations. Aveda's Exfoliant Liquid, Elemis' Skin Buff, Origins' Starting Over, Guerlain's Les Gestes Pûreté Radiant Gentle Exfoliator and Remède's Sweep are all gentle exfoliants.

To tone or not to tone?

First came the toner, and now there's the astringent, the skin freshener and the clarifying lotion, not forgetting the simple splash of water which, if you've cleansed your face thoroughly, will tone it as well as any fancy bottled product. Indeed, some facialists believe that buying a toner is the equivalent of pouring money down the drain. Eve Lom's cost-free method of toning is to cover your face with a muslin face cloth that has been run under the cold tap – simple it may be, but it works. A toner will leave your skin slightly damp, which can help moisturiser glide on more easily. For those whose cleansing technique is rather slapdash, a wipe-over with toner will ensure that every scrap of cleanser is removed. But, contrary to any convincing wording, no toner can actually close your pores.

Unless you have particularly tough, oily skin, alcohol-based astringents should be avoided as they are too harsh and will imbalance the skin's acid mantle. A word of advice: if you want to use a toner, tissue off any remnants or it could dehydrate your skin. For those who love that fresh, clean feeling that a toner gives you, a few toners that are kind to your skin include: Clarins' Extra Comfort Toning Lotion, The Body Shop's Cucumber Water, E'spa's Herbal Spa Fresh and Borghese's Spa Soothing Tonic. You can also make a DIY toner (see page 164).

Nourish and protect

Perhaps the most perplexing of all cosmetic products, in terms of the claims made for and against it, is the face cream. The good news is that moisturisers are at last beginning to meet the targets that they have proclaimed: protecting your face from environmental damage, nourishing your skin, preserving its water content and, because of all this, slowing down the ageing process. Every skin type (even oily skin) needs some form of moisturiser to help to replace lost moisture and protect it from the elements. Here are a few old and new favourites: Synergie's Vitamin Radiance Daily Moisturising Fluid, Kiehl's Ultra Facial Moisturiser, Karin Herzog's Vit-A-Kombi cream, Clinique's Turnaround Cream, Oil of Ulay's Active Beauty Fluid, Revlon's Eterna 27+ Instant-wonder Cream and Prescriptives' All You Need.

Night-time repair

Are night creams really worth their cost or the extra shelf space? Because scientists have now proved that the rate of the skin's cell production doubles when we are sleeping, it seems logical that we should be encouraging this renewal process by using a good cream, be it a night cream, day cream or a regular moisturiser. The advantage of applying a specially formulated night cream is that it has been developed to help promote optimum cell function. That having said, however, some facialists believe that your skin needs to breathe at night. Indeed, it's worth noting that while we are sleeping the skin rids itself of toxins; over moisturising will block the pores and prevent it from breathing, so if you do use a night cream only apply a thin film. Three good night creams include Origins' Night-A-Mins, Lancôme's Primordiale Nuit and Lancaster's Skin Therapy Oxygen For Night.

Treatments and serums

Cosmetics companies have created certain products that promise to encourage cellular repair, step up collagen production, and help strengthen and firm the skin. They may not be miracles in a jar, but these treatments do work that little bit harder conditioning your face than your usual moisturiser. Some can be used continuously, but many should simply be reserved as a treat for your skin when it is dry and thirsty for moisture. In order to give your face a mega-conditioning boost, invest in a serum or treatment such as: Ingrid Millet's Perle de Caviar Bio Marine Extract, Jo Malone's Protein Skin Serum, Elizabeth Arden's Skin Illuminating Complex, Dior's Capture Essentiel Time-fighting Serum, Avon's Stress Shield, La Prairie's Age Management Intensified Serum or Guerlain's Issima Midnight Secret Treatment.

Masks

Whether you want to deep cleanse your face or rehydrate it with a moisturising mask, your skin will really benefit from a weekly mask. Other kinds of masks include those formulated to firm or give instant radiance. Before using one, you should first assess the condition of your skin in order to ascertain which kind you need. Those with combination skin, for instance, may want to apply two different types: a deep-cleansing mask on the T-zone, such as Philosophy's Stuck in the Mud Clay Mask, and a moisturising mask on the cheeks, like Caudalie's Revitalising Moisture Grape-seed Cream Mask.

SKIN PROBLEMS AND SOLUTIONS

One of the biggest beauty headaches is problem skin so, if you are
suffering from breakouts, excessively dry or upset skin, here are a number of solutions to
help you return badly behaved skin to normal.

DRY, FLAKY SKIN

Excessively dry skin that feels rough and may even flake or peel, can be caused by cold weather, central heating or may simply occur because the sebaceous glands are not producing enough oil.

Treatment As water can be dehydrating, using a thick, wipe-off cleansing cream, lotion or milk is preferable to the less rich facial washes and cleansing bars. Exfoliate regularly, and after cleansing, nourish skin with a rich moisturiser: try products from ranges that have been specially formulated for dry skin, such as Helena Rubinstein's H^2O and Dior's Hydra Star. Consider treating your skin to a special-treatment serum, vitamin-E oil or a moisturising mask. Furthermore, ensure you drink plenty of water and lubricate your skin from within by sprinkling vegetable oils (which contain essential fatty acids) on salads, eating plenty of oily fish and taking such supplements as evening-primrose, borage or cod-liver oil.

OILY SKIN

'You won't age so quickly,' the beautician reassured me, but at that time I would rather have had wrinkles than every pore oozing grease. Oily skin is the result of increased sebum production, which can clog the pores and lead to blackheads and spots.

Treatment Steer clear of fatty or sugary foods, drink plenty of water, and eat a diet that is rich in vitamin B, which will help to slow down the skin's oil-production rate. Don't be tempted to use harsh, alcohol-based or medicated products on your skin, as these exacerbate the problem by stripping away the skin's natural oils and upsetting its pH balance. Instead, use a gentle product from the plethora of skincare ranges available that have been specially formulated to control oil by balancing the skin: try Aveda's Balancing Infusion for oily skin, Swisscare Givenchy's Regulating range or Clarins' Oil Control range, for example. If you feel the need to wash your face more often than just in the morning and at night, this is fine, as long as you only do so once, because overwashing can produce more oil.

The skin's natural oils act as a lubricant, but oily skin also needs moisture to help it to lock in water and prevent dehydration – it's not uncommon for skin to be oily and dehydrated at the same time. Compromise by using a light, oil-free moisturiser, such as Philosophy's The Present Oil-Free, Clinique's Moisture In Control Oil-Free Lotion or L'Oréal's Plenitude Hydra-Matify All Day Shine Control Moisturiser. If you wear foundation, choose a mattifying, oil-free formulation, such as Almay's Clear Balance Foundation or compact, Bobbi Brown's Oil Free Foundation, YSL's Teint Mat Parfait or Mabelline's Oil Free Foundation. Finally, a dab of an oil-control product, such as Lancôme's T-contrôle or Origins' Zero Oil, will mop up any excess oil and keep your face shine-free.

UPSET SKIN

Such varied factors as stress, fatigue, hormones, cosmetic-product overload, drugs, washing powder, caffeine, alcohol, illness, climatic change and certain foods can play havoc with your skin, causing it to become sensitive. According to dermatologists, as many

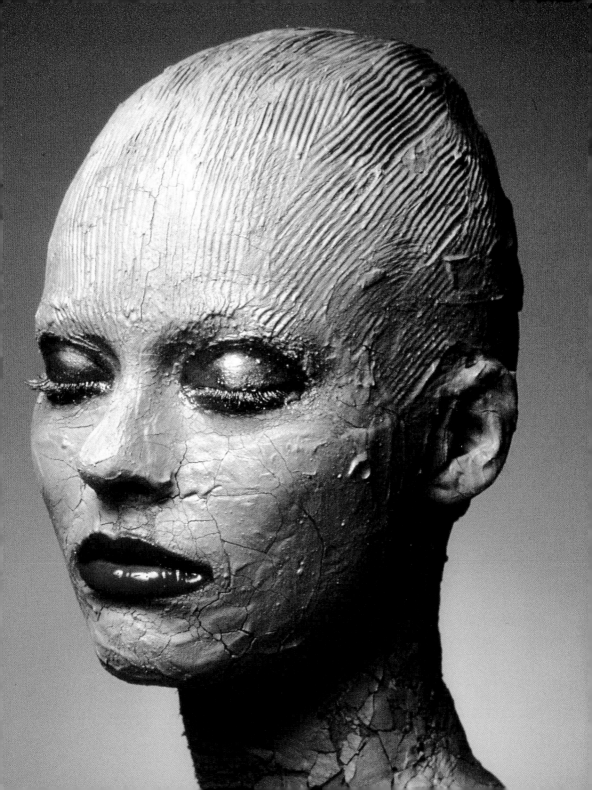

as eighty per cent of women complain of red, itchy and inflamed skin, but with a little care and the right products, such skin can be calmed down and desensitised.

Treatment Try using preparations based on natural ingredients or products designed for sensitive skin, such as Aveda's All Sensitive range, Estée Lauder's Verite range, Clinique's Exceptionally Soothing Lotion For Upset Skin or Johnson's pH 5.5 range. If your skin suddenly flares up, use nothing but aqueous cream – a basic cream that dermatologists recommend for cleansing and moisturising ultra sensitive skin which is available from pharmacies. If you are product-sensitive, always patch-test a preparation for at least three days and avoid such irritants as AHAs and highly fragranced products.

CONFUSED SKIN

Your T-zone (forehead, nose and chin) is greasy yet your cheeks are on the dry side – sound familiar? Combination skin plagues many of us from time to time, but because we are dealing with two conflicting problems we rarely get it right, tending either to dehydrate the dry zones further or to accelerate sebum production in the oily areas even more.

Treatment Don't treat your skin as if it is oily: ideally, you should use gentle, balancing products that control the oily areas yet keep the rest of the face well moisturised, such as YSL's Visiblé Energie For Combination Skin, La Prairie's Cellular Balancing Complex, Virgin Vie's Well-adjusted For Confused and Superficially Dehydrated Skin or Vichy's Adaptive Skin Balancing System Moisturiser.

SPOTS AND ACNE

Anyone who has ever suffered from acne will know that having a face full of spots is depressing and demoralising. Contrary to popular perception, this common skin condition doesn't only affect teenagers: acne can flare up in the twenties, thirties and even during the menopause, triggered by stress and hormonal changes. If you have more than just a few spots, to prevent being left with permanent scars, seek help from your doctor or a dermatologist.

Treatment

- **Diet:** rethink your diet. Start by avoid fatty and sugary foods, citrus fruits, caffeine and alcohol. Drink plenty of water, eat garlic and onions (for their antibacterial properties) and high-fibre food (to prevent a sluggish digestive system).

- **Skincare:** keep your skin scrupulously clean and do not squeeze spots (unless they are ready to burst). Avoid overusing antibacterial products and spot remedies containing alcohol or hydrocortisone, because if the surface of the skin dries out, sebum will become trapped and the acne could get worse. Instead, use a gentle spot zapper. Try to leave your skin free to breathe, concealing only the spots and scars. If you must wear base, use a powder-based or oil-free foundation.

- **Natural remedies:** herbal and homeopathic remedies can be effective in treating mild acne. Natural supplements that are known to help acne include evening-primrose oil (to help balance hormones); echinacea, propolis, burdock, purple cornflower, vitamin C and zinc (to help fight infection); and vitamin B (to slow down the rate of oil production).

- **Other treatments:** acne which has been caused by a hormonal imbalance can respond positively to certain types of contraceptive pill such as Dianette. The vitamin-A-derived oral drug Roaccutane is claimed to cure acne permanently in as many as seventy per cent of cases. However, due to the risk of side effects – including extremely dry, flaky skin and liver damage – it is only used as a last resort to treat serious conditions. Antibiotics tackle acne superficially but, as they only suppress the problem rather than cure it, the spots normally return once the patient has stopped taking the drugs. Topical antibiotic lotions are an alternative, albeit temporary, solution. The topical vitamin-A derivative, Retin-A, which is also used to reverse sun damage, was originally used to treat acne. But, because it can cause peeling and irritation, some dermatologists are now reluctant to prescribe it for acne.

ECZEMA

This itchy, inflammatory skin condition can affect people of all ages and is often hereditary. Eczema looks like just a dry patch of skin, but as the skin is usually red, scaly and uncomfortably itchy – and in acute cases, blistered or weeping – it can prematurely age the skin and cause discomfort to the sufferer. It is not contagious, although skin can become infected through scratching. There are several forms of eczema, but they generally fall into two main types. The first stems from within, and is triggered by such factors as a poor immune system, a bad diet or stress. The second is known as contact eczema (or dermatitis), which is the result of the skin having come into contact with detergents, soap, jewellery or another irritant.

Treatment If you think that you have contact eczema, carry out a patch test on the substance that you suspect might be the culprit; testing for any intolerance to food may also identify those that aggravate the condition. As far as skincare products are concerned, use ranges based on natural ingredients and, unless the condition is severe, avoid using steroid creams as these thin the skin (although the new non-steroid creams are a promising alternative). If eczema is affecting your body, try soaking in a bath with healing minerals, such as Dead Sea salts. Eczema-improving natural supplements include evening-primrose or borage oil, vitamin A, zinc and burdock.

ACNE SCARS

There are two types of acne scar. The first is the reddish, purplish mark that remains after the spot has healed; unless the capillaries have become permanently dilated, most of these marks should eventually fade in time. Pitting is the second, and more severe form of scarring, and is usually the aftermath of large spots and boils. These permanent scars, take the shape of crater-like holes in the skin, which are not dissimilar to chicken-pox scars.

Treatment Minimise any reddish scarring by applying vitamin-E oil or a calamine-based product. When taken orally, vitamin-B complex or arnica can help to speed up the healing process. As the skin renews itself, most pitted scars become less obvious in time, but they are occasionally so deep that skin resurfacing (using laser or chemical peels) is the only solution (see page 103). Superficial skin peels or using a Retin-A preparation can mildly improve the appearance of both types of scar.

BLACKHEADS

Blackheads are little plugs of sebum that are trapped in the pores; their black tops are not dirt, but are instead caused by the sebum's oxidation on its exposure to air.

Treatment Blackheads can be removed with a blackhead extractor or by using your fingers (wrapped in a tissue), but the recent invention of such blackhead strips as Bioré's Pore-cleansing Strips for the face and nose or Ponds Clear Pore Strips, have made their removal both quicker and kinder to your skin. A Retin-A preparation can also help the problem. If you want your blackhead evacuation to be carried out by a professional, go to a good beauty salon for a deep-cleansing facial, such as Guinot's Catheodermie, or a vacuum-suction facial which hoovers the blackheads into a tube.

WHITEHEADS

Whiteheads are white bumps under the skin (known as milia), which can persist for long periods of time. They consist of trapped sebum that started out as a liquid substance before eventually becoming hard and waxy. A more common form of whitehead are the tiny lumps which can accumulate around the eye zone.

Treatment Whiteheads are far more difficult to remove than blackheads. One way of tackling them is to disperse them with gentle massage as soon as they appear. Don't try to extract them yourself, for if you end up pushing them deeper into the pores they could result in nasty spots. If the whitehead is too stubborn for a beauty therapist to extract, a dermatologist can dry it up by injecting it with cortisone.

THE BODY BEAUTIFUL

Bare-minimum fashions demand a perfectly smooth, blemish-free and gleaming body – here's how to achieve it.

Few of us are ever content with our bodies – even supermodels grumble about their bodily blips – yet most of us neglect our bodies by adopting the out-of-sight, out-of-mind attitude, that is until the time comes to cast off our clothes and don our bikinis: only then when we have to reveal our bodies do we realise that it's too late for miracle diets or anti-cellulite strategies.

IMPROVE YOUR SKIN

Having to face the world with dry, dimpled skin is bad enough, but the thought of svelte Baywatch-style babes in incy wincy bikinis, is enough to make most of us break out in a cold sweat. But before you start loathing the warm weather just because it's too hot to wear those concealing woolly jumpers and tights, take heart: with a little sloughing and softening you can improve your body in a matter of weeks.

Body Polish

Dead skin cells tend to accumulate on the skin, especially on neglected parts of your body, like your back. If you've ever scratched your back and come away with fingernails full of dirt, you'll know what I mean. Thankfully, the appearance of dry and pasty-looking skin can be improved almost immediately by exfoliating, which is also an effective way to prepare your skin to be more receptive to body lotion.

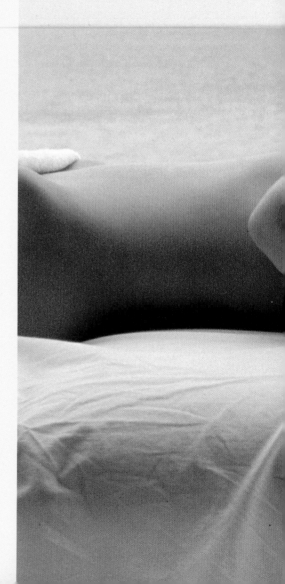

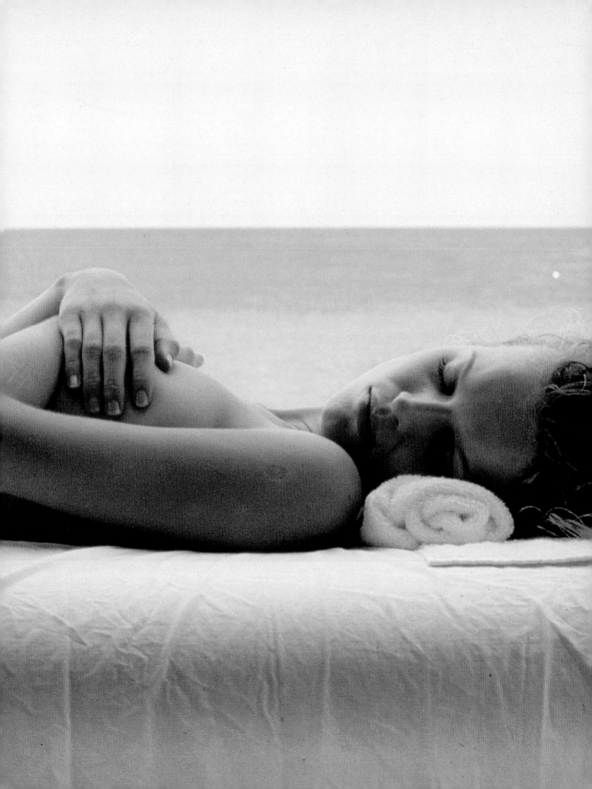

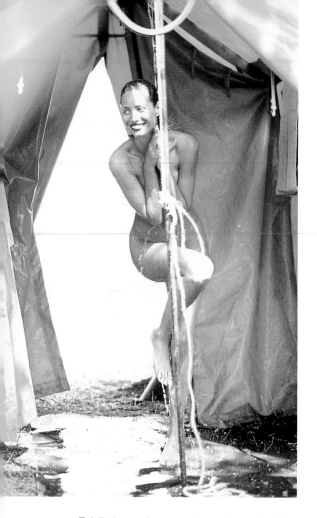

Have baby-soft skin

A soft, smooth, silky skin does wonders for your confidence, but if the last time that you slathered on body lotion was after a day's roasting on the beach, your body is probably crying out – and drying out – for moisture. The skin on our bodies contains fewer sebaceous glands than that of the face, which means that it produces less natural oil. So if you want to avoid dry, crepy skin, it is vital that you moisturise daily.

Bodycare products have now become as sophisticated as those for the face, with many cosmetics companies using the same 'wonder' ingredients found in face creams to help to improve the texture of the skin and guard against ageing. These are a few of the most popular body moisturisers, ranging from the inexpensive ones that you'll find in the supermarket, to the most luxurious designer lotions: Revlon's Dry Skin Relief, Neutrogena's Daily Moisture Supply, Bharti Vyas' Body Lotion, Helena Rubinstein's Force-C Body Mousse, Vaseline's Intensive Care Body Lotion and Donna Karan's Cashmere Body Lotion. For extra-dry or callused areas, try Eve Lom's TLC, Gatineau's Vigoceane Moisturising Lotion, Vaseline Petroleum Jelly or Kiehl's Intensive Moisturiser. In order to lock the maximum amount of moisture into your skin, apply liberal amounts of lotion to damp skin.

Better your skin tone

The skin on your body, like that on your face, loses its elasticity with time. Although a cream may claim to firm up your body, only exercise can effectively tone the muscles. However, refining, toning, lifting and firming creams and lotions can improve the appearance of the skin and make it feel more supple, especially if you combine their application with the three pronged attack of firm massage, skin-brushing and exercise. These are just some of the many firming creams on the market: Dior's Svelte Perfect, Clarins' Lift-Minceur Body Lift, Shiseido's Essential Energy Body Firming Cream and Decleor's System Corps Moisturising and Firming Emulsion. Spend as long as possible massaging cream into your skin – especially on thighs, buttocks and upper arms, as this will improve skin tone.

Exfoliating actions can be performed either on dry skin, using a towel, mitt or loofah or, alternatively, on wet skin whilst showering with one of the dozens of body scrubs available, such as The Body Shop's Marmalade Scrub or Clarins' Exfoliating Body Scrub. If you don't have a body scrub, try a health-spa favourite: a handful of finely ground sea salt, or turn to page 164 for other DIY scrubs. Massage your exfoliator into damp skin, working in light, circular movements all over your body, paying particular attention to such hard-skin zones as the elbows, knees and soles of feet. And don't forget your hands, they really benefit from regular exfoliation. Always apply a body lotion afterwards.

Be a bathing beauty

Not so long ago, a soak in a bath filled with pretty coloured, scented bubbles was deemed enough to relax you, although the product did little to benefit your skin. With today's dizzying array of first-class bathing preparations on the market, however, you can both condition your skin and transform your basic bath-time ablutions into a spa experience: you can bathe in algae, sprinkle mineral salts in to your bath or relax with aromatherapy oils. Beauty guru Bharti Vyas is a great believer in bathing in Dead Sea salts: 'The salts contain a high concentration of minerals, which benefit both the skin and body.' While a long soak in a bath is a luxury, a shower is more of an everyday occurrence. Whenever you shower, become tingly fresh with a good, moisturising body wash or shower gel, but avoid soap as this will sap your body's moisture.

Keep your back blemish free

If you have a congested, spotty back, shower emollients containing antibacterial agents, such as The Body Shop's Tea-tree Oil Body Wash or Kiehl's Tea-tree Oil Body Wash, will help tackle the problem. Exfoliate regularly using a gentle body scrub and light movements so as not to aggravate the problem. Allow skin to breathe by wearing loose clothing. If you can hardly put a pin between your spots, you will need some form of treatment for acne, so seek your doctor's advice (see page 124 for details of treatments).

Skin-brush daily

Skin-brushing may seem to be yet another ritual that means having to get out of bed even earlier, but just a couple of minutes a day spent brushing your skin really pays off. Regular brushing with a dry brush before your bath or shower does more than simply buff away dead cells: it cleanses the pores while smoothing, toning and firming the skin. Beauty benefits aside, it stimulates blood circulation, boosts the flow of nutrients to the skin and encourages lymphatic drainage. Using a relatively firm, dry, natural-bristle body brush, start at your feet and work up your body, using sweeping movements always towards the direction of your heart.

DE-FUZZ YOUR BODY

Unless a hairy body turns you or your partner on, it is essential to remove unwanted hair for a feminine, well-groomed look and smooth skin. These are some of the main methods of hair removal. **Shaving** is the quickest way in which to remove hair, yet it is the most temporary by far, as stubble tends to sprout the following day. You may prefer to use a specially angled razor, which is less likely to nick or cut your skin. Shaving is only suitable for the underarms and legs, not the bikini line or face. **Depilatory creams** can be used at home and are an easy, albeit rather messy, form of hair removal. You apply the cream to the hairy zone, wait for a few minutes and then rinse it off. These creams can be used on most areas, although there are specially formulated ones for the face. **Epilators** whip out the hair at the roots. There is no regrowth for a couple of weeks. **Waxing** uses either hot or cold wax which is applied to the hairy area before being stripped off a few minutes later. Ouch! It's a touch painful, but the hair-free results last for at least two weeks. **Electrolysis** which involved the use of a needle has been superseded by Transdermal electrolysis. Using a probe-like instrument and conducting gel, a galvanic current is sent directly to the root of the hair to destroy it. Suitable for most areas, the major advantage of this form of electrolysis is its long-lasting results; as each hair needs to be individually treated, however, many visits to the salon are needed before you are hair-free. **Bleaching** can be carried out on most body hair, but is particularly effective on the fine, down-like facial hair. You can buy DIY home-bleaching kits or have it done professionally. **Sugaring** is an age-old, Eastern form of hair removal that has now become popular in the West. Carried out either at home with a DIY kit or at a beauty salon, sugaring removes hair in much the same way as waxing: the sugar paste is applied to the area and then stripped off. Regrowth is not visible for two weeks. **Scanning** uses a high-intensity frequency to remove hairs. You can have unwanted hair removed from the face and body permanently using a form of **laser** known as the Epilaser.

SHIFT CELLULITE

It's lumpy, bumpy and looks like orange peel. We all dread it, yet the majority of us suffer from this unsightly, hard-to-shift condition on our bottoms, thighs and upper arms. Caused by a combination of factors, such as bad diet, poor circulation, sluggish digestion, fluid retention, lack of exercise and the female hormone oestrogen, no matter how slim you are, you can still be a victim of cellulite. What causes the dimpling effect are fatty deposits protruding through weakened connective tissue, which manifest themselves as lumpy, raised areas. No single diet, treatment, exercise or anti-cellulite cream will combat cellulite alone, but if you eat healthily, exercise and persevere with massage and skin-brushing, you can certainly go some way to improve it.

Home treatments for cellulite
Massage: by boosting the circulation and encouraging drainage, massage can help to disperse fatty deposits. **Diet:** eat a healthy, balanced, high-fibre, low-fat diet and drink plenty of water. Vitamin E and C supplements can help to get rid of cellulite. Cut down on tea, coffee and alcohol, and avoid sugary, salty, smoked and spicy foods. **Exercise:** flexibility exercises, such as body-stretching or yoga, stretch the leg tissues and encourage fluid movement. **Water therapy:** if you have a power-shower, bursts of cold water interspersed with warm directed on to the cellulite zone is another way of decongesting cellulite. **Skin-brushing** your body daily will rev up your circulation and tone the skin, making it appear firmer. **Anti-cellulite creams** can help to strengthen the skin's surface and make the flesh appear smoother, but they cannot banish cellulite. Some of the good ones include Dior's Svelte Perfect, Lancaster's Recontour Anti-cellulite Gel, Decleor's Cellulium, Borghese's Supple Body Contour (with a built-in massage applicator), Kanebo's Cosmetic Body Sash and Serum For Thighs, or Tisserand's Cellulite Gift Pack (which includes essential oils and a wooden massager). **Electronic toners** for home use, such as Philip's Cellese, have the same effect as massage and are great for those who are too busy or just lazy.

Salon or surgical treatments for cellulite
Salon treatments: detoxifying body wraps or treatments, such as Ionithermie, fibreoptic light therapy, Endermologie or C.A.C.I., which use an electrical current or ultrasound, can improve cellulite. However, it often takes a course of ten sessions before you see any results. **Medical treatments:** mesotherapy – injections of drugs to help drain away excess fluid – can reduce cellulite. Another method is cellulolipolysis, in which needles are attached to electrodes and inserted under the skin. **Surgical treatments:** liposuction is a rather radical method of removing cellulite and not always successful.

PREVENT STRETCHMARKS

If parts of your body – in particular your thighs, bottom and breasts – resemble a road map, you are probably already a victim of stretchmarks. Once you have them, there is no simple cure, however. Often caused by fluctuating weight or an increase in breast and stomach size during pregnancy, even the laser can't zap away the stubborn ones. You can nevertheless prevent the formation of stretchmarks and, if you catch them early enough, stop them in their tracks. Work at softening them and preventing them from becoming worse by keeping vulnerable areas moisturised with vitamin-E oil, apricot-kernel oil, or a cream like Eve Lom's Crème Universelle or Gatineau's Vergeturia Suractivee Restructuring Cream.

Retin-A preparations can help eliminate any redness and smooth the skin, while the Ebrium-Yag laser can obliterate minor stretchmarks and improve deeper ones by regenerating the skin.

LOVE YOUR LEGS

A smooth, silky pair of legs is a great physical attribute, so start tackling rough areas, such as knees and heels, by exfoliating and moisturising them; your daily routine should also include skin-brushing. If you tend to sit at your desk with your legs crossed you are committing the biggest leg-beauty crime of all, for this blocks circulation and encourages thread veins and cellulite to torment your legs. Puffy legs respond well to a salon treatment known as Flowtron – inflatable leggings which, by applying pressure to the lymphatic points, encourage drainage. Finally, for legs that look a little pasty, apply self-tan.

FIRM UP YOUR BUST

Breasts do not contain any muscular tissue, but because they are supported by the chest's pectoral muscles, you can firm them up to some extent by exercising (see Radu's exercises for breasts). Salon treatments for the bust, such as those offered by Clarins, Decleor, Cathiodermie, Thalgo and Ionithermie, will improve your bust's appearance, but the results are only temporary. There are also creams and toning lotions available which, although they cannot lift the bust or change its shape, can keep the surrounding skin supple and smooth. You can even tone up your breasts for free by simply splashing them with cold water. Maintaining your bust's health includes checking your posture, wearing a good, supportive bra and being measured every six months to check whether your bra size has altered.

TACKLE YOUR VEINS

A century ago, women would draw veins on their bodies as transparent skin was viewed as a sign of youth. Sadly, these days veins are categorised as yet another bodily imperfection. Tiny thread veins (also known as spider veins) can be found on your body, as well as your face, and are due to loss of elasticity in the capillary wall, which causes them to dilate. Veins are tricky to disguise and even the deepest-golden tan will do little to hide them. However, you could try covering them with a camouflage product like Dermablend's Cover Cream or a waterproof or long-lasting foundation, such as Revlon's ColorStay. Vitamin K-based creams are said to improve the appearance of thread veins. For permanent removal, there are opitons such as micro-sclerotherapy, electrolysis, or having them zapped with a laser.

DON'T NEGLECT YOUR NECK AND DECOLLETAGE

Just like the face, the neck is constantly on show, yet we scarcely give it any attention. But according to dermatologist Dr Catherine Orentreich, the neck is an area that is resistant to cosmetic intervention, so looking after it and shielding it with a sunscreen is vitally important. Crepiness is a sign of both dehydration and dead skin cells clinging to the skin's surface. So if you want to keep your neck silky smooth and young looking, you need to extend your full skincare routine to it and, because the skin contains less sebum here, apply a rich cream twice daily.

Your décolletage is that sensual area that lies between your bust and neck, yet even the the sexiest cleavage will be spoilt if this area is marred by lines. Sun damage and the way in which you sleep are the primary thieves that can rob you of a smooth, line-free décolletage. As it is always the first area to burn when you are sunbathing, make sure that you protect it. And because the skin is thinner here than on other parts of the body, unless you lie on your back when you are sleeping, it becomes folded and creased. In order to prevent the formation of lines and crease marks, always moisturise your décolletage during the day and use a barrier cream such as Vaseline Petroleum Jelly at night.

A SUN-KISSED BODY

A deep-golden tan makes you look slimmer, healthier and twice
as sexy. But, as exposing your body to the sun is a cardinal beauty sin, play it safe by
following this sun-survival guide.

Bright-blue skies, long, hot summer days and the glorious feeling of warm sunshine beating down on you – there's nothing quite like it. Sunshine is undoubtedly a great mood-enhancer and, if taken in small doses, exposing our bodies to the sun can be beneficial: sunlight stimulates the body's production of vitamin D, which helps us to absorb calcium. However, exposure to the sun triggers melanin production – the body's protective mechanism; this turns us brown but with detrimental effects. It's a well-documented fact that the sun causes ninety per cent of all wrinkles, not to mention ugly brown spots and skin cancer. It therefore seems as though we are sacrificing an awful lot for the sake of a bit of colour, especially now that we can achieve the same sun-kissed look from a bottle.

The sun produces two forms of ultraviolet radiation: UVA and UVB. UVA rays cause the signs of ageing and increase the risk of skin cancer, while UVB rays burn the skin. The level of the sun-protection factor (SPF) contained in products designed to defend against UVB rays is determined by an SPF rating (the higher the number, the greater the protection), whereas UVA protection is indicated by star (***) ratings. Leading dermatologist Professor Nicholas Lowe believes that we should all be wearing a sunscreen with a SPF 15 on our faces every day. 'The sunscreen should have a three *** or four **** UVA star rating,' he adds. 'In the summer, on a day spent outdoors, or while snow-skiing in the winter, use a waterproof screen with an SPF of 25 to 30.' Professor Lowe recommends sunscreens by Ambre Solaire, Neutrogena, Nivea, Piz Buin, Soltan, Uvistat and Vaseline.

TIPS ON TANNING

- When choosing a sunscreen, look for one that offers protection against both UVAs and UVBs. Apply the lotion before you don your swimming costume and reapply generous amounts of it at hourly intervals throughout the day, and always after swimming. Start with a high protection factor of at least SPF 15, only using a lower number once you have built up a good base colour. Pay extra attention to zones that are prone to burning, such as your nose, lips, décolletage, breasts, knees and feet. Keep the lotion in the shade and discard it after two years.
- Be realistic about your ability to tan: if you have fair skin and freckles you are never going to achieve the same deep colour as those with olive skin.
- Always avoid exposure to the midday sun (that is, between the hours of eleven in the morning and three in the afternoon). Get some respite from the sun by retreating into the shade at regular intervals.
- If you are prone to acne, piling on rich sunscreens can make it worse. Look for sunscreens that have been specially formulated for the face that are light and non-comedogenic so that they won't block your pores.
- Whether you are walking, playing sport or sunbathing, you should wear a sun-protection cream and keep your head covered with a hat or scarf in order to prevent sunstroke or a burnt scalp. And if you are sailing or doing any other watersports, wear a water-resistant sunscreen; choose from a sports range that has a higher level of water resistance.

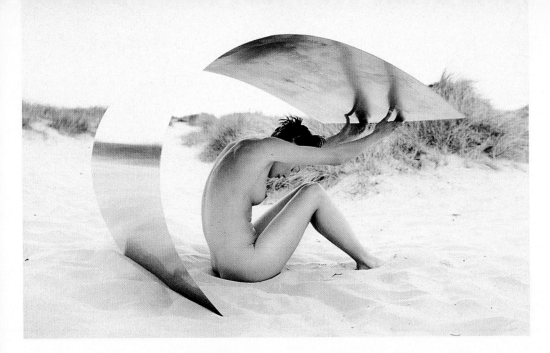

• The sea or pool may seem the perfect place in which to cool off, but remember that the sun's rays still penetrate water.

• Invest in a good pair of sunglasses to prevent you from squinting and protect your eyes from ultraviolet rays, which can cause cataracts and damage the eye's cornea and lens.

• Sunbeds and tanning units are just as harmful as the sun: although they rarely burn the skin, high-powered sunbeds and tanning units deliver highly concentrated amounts of ultraviolet light.

TIPS ON SELF-TANNING

The only safe route to acquire a tan is to fake it. The days when fake tan was orange-tinged, streaky and smelt of chemicals have long gone: today's formulations are so sophisticated that no one can tell the difference between a tan from a bottle or the sun; they also come in different shades to suit your skin tone. A great, all-over, golden tan is simple to achieve – the products are easy to apply, fast-drying and, if you apply them carefully, won't appear patchy. Follow these tips, or have a tanning product applied at a beauty salon, and between two to four hours later you'll have a gorgeous, golden tan that gradually fades in the course of a few days.

• For an even, streak-free tan, prime your body by exfoliating and moisturising it before applying the fake tan. Now massage the self-tanning lotion into your skin, using sweeping movements. To avoid build-up and obvious lines, apply it with great care to, and around, areas like your hairline, jaw, eyebrows, knees and ankles.

• If you make a mistake, fade-away products can banish any marks. Alternatively, try rubbing the area with a little toothpaste.

• For mess-free application and those difficult-to-reach spots, opt for a spray-on tan or ask a friend to apply the lotion for you.

• Allow thirty minutes for the lotion to dry and then wear loose clothes for at least an hour.

• If it's a deep tan that you are after, repeat the application (but wait for a few hours to ensure that the first layer has dried).

• Try one of the following products: Clinique's Self Sun Self Tanning Body Balm, St Tropez's Self Tan, Lancaster's Precise Ccolour Self Tan SPF 6, Ecotan's Self Tanning Spray, Ambre Solaire's Duo Tan Self Tanning Milk or RoC's Self Tanning Lotion SPF 6.

MARVELLOUS MITTS

Your hands are permanently on show, and while well-groomed, smooth hands with manicured nails are a prized asset, dry, wrinkled hands with chewed stumps for nails are one of the most noticeable signs of age and neglect.

SUPERHINTS FOR LOVELIER HANDS

- If you are washing up or handling detergent or any other chemical substance, wear rubber gloves (models wear gloves even when shampooing their hair).
- Always apply hand cream after washing your hands and whenever they look dry. Keep a tub of hand cream by your kitchen sink and bathroom basin to remind you to do this, and carry a tube in your handbag. Good hand creams include L'Occitane's Shea Butter, Jurlique's Lavender Hand Cream, Neutrogena's Norwegian Formula, Nivea's Hand Age Control Lotion and Vaseline's Intensive Care Hand Cream.
- For parched hands that are in desperate need of attention, try this overnight treatment and witness the difference in the morning. Massage your hands with a little warm olive or almond oil and pop them into cotton gloves that have been warmed on a radiator; a moisturising face mask or even hand cream will also do the trick. For a real treat, try Borghese's Moisture Restoring Gloves or Mavela's Night Cream For Hands.
- Exfoliate your hands regularly, using either a mixture of finely-ground sea salt and glycerine, your body or face exfoliator or a tailor-made product for hands, such as Philosophy's Time On Your Hands – a cream and exfoliator in one.
- If your hands have brown marks (caused by the sun or ageing), RoC's Retinol Anti-ageing Hand Cream and Cellex-C's Salacia Lotion can help these spots to fade away. The more stuborn ones respond well to laser treatment.
- Wear a sunscreen to protect your hands.

TALON TIPS

The condition of your nails is affected by your health and lifestyle. If your nails are healthy, they should be pink, strong and flexible, whereas unhealthy nails are brittle, yellow in colour, often have ridges, and flake, split and break easily. Many nail problems are caused by vitamin and mineral deficiencies, so start by taking a good multi-vitamin-and-mineral supplement and eat a well-balanced diet.

- Shorter nails are more fashionable at the moment and, as well as being easier to maintain, are less likely to split than long talons.
- If you can't be bothered with nail varnish, or prefer wearing your nails nude, use a nail buffer to smooth the surface of you nails, even out any ridges and give your nails a natural gloss.
- In order to boost your nails' blood circulation and encourage healthy growth, using your thumb, massage the nail bed daily with a little olive oil, nail oil or a nail-strengthening cream.
- Prevent your nails from tearing by being extra careful when handling or opening zips, buttons, doors, cans and so on. If a nail does tear or split don't rip it off: repair kits and nail bandages are now available that can patch up or glue the nail back together again.
- Wear gloves to protect your nails while washing up or using detergents.
- If you nibble your nails, the only way in which to get them to look halfway decent is to wear false ones. You can have tips built onto them by a manicurist, or build your own using one of the false-nail kits available like Elegant Touch's Ultra-quick Gel Nail Kit or Nailene's Acrylic Kit Salon Sculpting System.

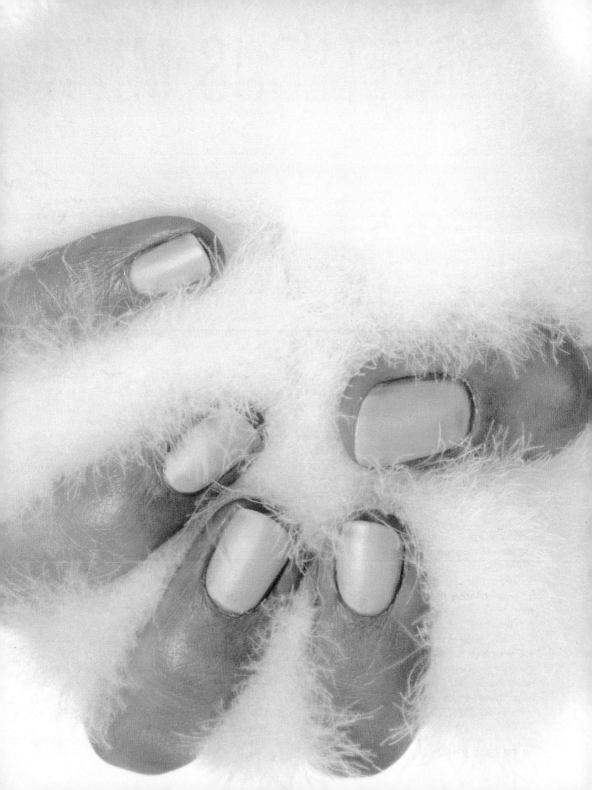

POLISH UP

Whether you prefer subtle shades or in-your-face cherry-black, varnished nails will give the final touch to your total look; nail polish also acts as protection. Colour makes a dramatic difference to nails, so if you've got the guts – be bold. Here are a few tips to help your nails reach a state of polished perfection.

• Create your own customised nail colour by layering on two differently coloured varnishes (you may want to experiment on paper first).

• It is quicker and easier to retouch chipped nail polish than to wipe it all off and start again. And, as nail-polish remover has a dehydrating effect, it is also kinder to your nails.

• Before applying polish, clean your nails with nail-polish remover to prevent any subsequent streaking or bubbles.

• Choose an acetone-free nail-polish remover as it is gentler and therefore less likely to dry out the horny, keratinous layer of the nail, or to cause brittle nails or splitting.

• Speed up the polish's drying time by using a quick-drying varnish or spray, such as Sally Hanson's Dry-fast Nail Spray, Opi's Rapidry Spray, Revlon's Top Speed Enamel or Maybelline's Express Finish Nail Polish. Plunging your fingers into cold water also works.

• If you end up with more polish on your finger than on the nail itself, there's no need to start again: simply dip a cotton bud in nail-polish remover and wipe off any blobs.

• For those who lack polish precision, nail beauty aids are now available, including stencils, transfers and complete-nail-shaped adhesives, which means that you can do away with polish altogether.

• Professional-looking French manicures can be achieved at home with the help of stencils or a white nail pencil.

• Using an undercoat or primer will stop bold colours staining your nails, while applying a nail-strengthening base will keep nails conditioned and fill in any ridges.

• Protect your nails and prevent them from chipping by applying a clear nail protector as a top coat.

NAIL ART

Nails decorated with gems, glitter and flowers have been regular fixtures on the catwalk. The Untouchables, the duo responsible for models' talons, are to nails what Sam McKnight and Mary Greenwell are to runway hair and make-up. Here are their tips for nail art. 'Do experiment with nail art, because it can be taken off as quickly as it can be put on. Choose a base colour that suits your skin tone rather than going straight for the colour that is in fashion. Simple additions to this base colour can be very effective, for example, a rhinestone on each nail or a daisy painted on the little fingernail. Adapt nail fashion to what suits you personally.'

HOME MANICURE

You will need: nail polish (including base, colour and top coat), an emery board, a nail buffer, a hand, face or body exfoliator, a cuticle remover, almond oil, nail-strengthening cream, nail oil or vegetable oil, a nail brush and cotton buds.

Step 1   Remove old nail polish or clean your nails with an acetone-free nail-polish remover.

Step 2   Using the coarse (darker) side of an emery board, shape your nails, working from the outer edge to the middle and filing in one direction only. Once shaped, smooth the edges of nails with the finer side of the emery board.

Step 3   Exfoliate hands with your face or body scrub, or a little salt mixed with glycerine.

Step 4   Soak nails in warm water to which a drop of almond oil has been added. Using a nail brush, gently scrub the underneath of your nails. Dry your hands thoroughly.

Step 5   Massage a drop of nail oil or nail-strengthening cream into each nail (if you don't possess either, olive or almond oil will also do). Now rub in a cuticle remover. Then, taking a cotton bud, gently push back the cuticles. Rinse your hands and dry them thoroughly.

Step 6   If you prefer your nails nude, use a buffer to smooth ridges and add sheen. To polish, start with a base coat followed by a second coat. Finally, paint on a clear top coat, which will protect the nail and seal in the colour.

FABULOUS FEET

We squeeze them into ill-fitting shoes, stand on them on for hours at a time and still expect them to look after themselves. But treat your feet to some tender loving care and you will have a pair to be proud of.

SUPERHINTS FOR PRETTY FEET

- Prevent the build-up of hard skin and calluses by exfoliating and buffing the soles of your feet with a pumice stone or foot file.
- When you apply your body lotion, remember to massage your feet (not forgetting the soles). Alternatively, purchase a good, antibacterial foot cream that will moisturise, refresh and protect your feet from fungal infections.
- Ill- or tight-fitting shoes and towerblock-like heels can make you feel miserable and put a strain on your ankles and back. So make sure that your shoes fit you correctly.
- Let your feet breathe by wearing sandals or going barefoot whenever possible. Replace nylon socks with cotton ones and wear cotton insoles in your shoes.
- Foot baths, sprays and powders will help to keep feet smelling sweet and also revive tired feet. If your foot odour knocks you backwards, beauty guru Bharti Vyas suggests that soaking feet in a salt bath (using Dead Sea salts) will correct the pH balance of the skin and help to make your feet smell sweet again.
- Be meticulous as regards foot hygiene. Always dry your feet thoroughly and use a foot powder. To avoid catching fungal infections, wear flip-flops in changing rooms and when walking beside a public swimming pool.
- Prevent any foot problems developing by regularly inspecting your soles, heels and between your toes. Note that corns, verrucas, athlete's foot, ingrown toenails and other problems should be treated by a chiropodist.

HOME PEDICURE

You will need: a foot-soaking solution, a pumice stone or foot file, scissors or a nail clipper, an emery board, a cuticle remover, cotton buds or a hoofer (a rubber-ended nail tool), almond oil, nail-polish remover, nail polish and a toe-separator or pieces of cotton wool.

Step 1 Soak your feet in a warm foot bath. A good DIY foot-soak solution consists of a tablespoon of Epsom or Dead Sea salts; a couple of drops of almond oil to soften the skin; and a drop or two of peppermint, rosemary or tea-tree essential oil to refresh and revive feet.

Step 2 Slough off any dead skin on the soles of your feet with a pumice stone or foot file.

Step 3 Clip or cut your toenails into a square shape (overrounding them can cause ingrown nails). File your toenails with the coarse side of an emery board until they are smooth.

Step 4 Apply a cuticle remover and massage it into the nail bed. Now gently push the cuticles back with a cotton bud or a hoofer.

Step 5 Smooth on some almond oil and then give your feet a well-earned massage, using kneading movements. Rinse your feet and wipe off any remaining traces of oil from toenails with nail-polish remover.

Step 6 Apply polish to your toenails – even if this is the one and only thing you do to your feet. If you wear sandals, varnish will show that you take care of your feet. To make polishing easier, separate toes with a toe-separator or pieces of cotton wool. As with a manicure, apply a base before the second and top coat.

COSMETIC SURGERY

Once upon a time there was an ordinary girl from Ohio who was not only without a date for the high-school prom, but had also been rejected as a cheerleader for simply not being pretty enough. Then she visited the plastic surgeon, not once, but twenty or so times, for a nip here and a tuck there, as well as two face-lifts, three eye operations, lip enlargement, two breast operations, four liposuction treatments, three chemical peels, dermabrasion and a few other procedures. Several years later she was, undeniably, a beautiful woman, but her face and body was no longer her own.

Cindy Jackson – who is said to have modelled herself on the Sindy doll – was lucky: fall into the hands of a charlatan and you could be scarred for life. You can indeed get fantastic results with cosmetic surgery, but because of the risks involved, all surgical procedures should be considered carefully. And don't think that cosmetic surgery will magically solve all your problems and make you a happy person, or resurrect your marriage: it is by no means a cure-all. You may recall the true-life story of a woman called The Bride of Wildenstein – no amount of surgery would keep her husband.

Before you embark on any surgical procedure, make sure that you find a reputable and highly qualified cosmetic surgeon: ask your doctor and contact any related professional associations for advice until you find a surgeon with whom you feel happy about leaving your appearance in his or her hands.

COSMETIC PROCEDURES

These are the latest methods used for the most popular cosmetic procedures, compiled with the help of one of the world's leading plastic surgeons, Mr Brian Coghlan. (For skin resurfacing, facial fillers and other more minor procedures see page 102.)

Face-lifts

The latest endoscopic face- and brow-lift has done away with the taut, giveaway sign of a face-lift and, according to Mr Coghlan, this method also reduces scarring. 'Using keyhole surgery, we reposition muscle and facial tissue in the face and brow area with a telescope,' he explains. 'This works well on women in their late thirties and forties who have facial sagging. But for more mature women, and those with excess, loose skin, a "skin-lift" is more effective.'

There are also several other face-lifting procedures. One of the most popular is the SMAS (subcutaneous muscles aponeurotic system) lift: 'The SMAS layer and the platsyma muscle in the neck are corrected,' explains Mr Coghlan. 'This takes the tension off the skin layer allowing excess skin to be removed, before lifting, stretching and stitching it to the ear area and along the hairline.' Performed under general anaesthetic, the recovery time after a face-lift is approximately two weeks. Depending on the scale of the face-lift and the area of the face lifted, swelling can last for several weeks.

Nose reshaping

It's not only Michael Jackson who has bought the nose of his choice: rhinoplasty is one of the most popular cosmetic procedures. The nose can be shortened, lengthened, built up or made smaller but, according to Mr Coghlan, nowadays the trend is towards adjusting the shape of the nose as opposed to making it smaller. Changes on the surgical front to what is termed 'open surgery', in which the skin is lifted up, have resulted in easier access for surgeons. 'Although the patient is left with a tiny, barely noticeable scar on the central strut, open surgery makes remoulding easier,' says Mr Coghlan. After undergoing a general anaesthetic, the patient must wear a plaster for seven to ten days. Any bruising and swelling should subside after a couple of weeks.

Ear pinning

Those who hate their sticking-out ears can have them pinned back by means of this fairly simple operation (otoplasty). This procedure involves stitching the ears back onto the head leaving no visible scarring. 'In most cases we reshape the cartilage framework of the ear, which involves having to make incisions behind the ears', says Mr Coghlan. Ear pinning can be carried out under local anaesthetic, after which the patient must wear bandages for one week.

Cheek and chin augmentations

Using preshaped implants made from collagen, bodily fat or synthetic, bone-like substances, surgeons can build up cheekbones. Chin augmentation (mentoplasty) involves implants being inserted under the chin or through the mouth to reshape a receding chin. 'One of the current implants being used is coral, as it is a natural fibre that closely matches bone,' says Mr Coghlan, who goes on to explain that as the implants are inserted through the mouth there is no visible scarring. This operation requires a general anaesthetic and patients must expect some swelling. If the implant has been inserted via the mouth, aftercare involves meticulous oral hygiene in order to prevent infection.

Breast enlargements and reductions

Breasts can be enlarged, as well as reduced or uplifted. With both of these procedures, surgical advancements have resulted in a reduction in the amount of visible scarring: 'Surgeons are making smaller and neater incisions. For example, on a minor breast reduction there would only be scarring around the nipple,' says Mr Coghlan. Despite the silicone scare, breast augmentation remains in demand. For the past eighteen months Mr Coghlan, along with many other surgeons, has been using Hydrogel: 'The shell, as with all breast implants, is silicone, but inside is a salty, sugary, water-like substance that will not cause problems if any leakage occurs.' After all types of breast surgery, which require a general anaesthetic, patients must wear a support bra for several weeks to help mould their breasts into shape.

Eye surgery

Droopy eyelids can benefit from upper-eyelid surgery (blepharoplasty). 'For this operation we need to make an incision which leaves a small, single scar line in the crease; this is not visible when the eyes are open', says Mr Coghlan. Lower-eye surgery removes or redeposits fat, but as it cannot eliminate crow's-feet, it is often combined with laser resurfacing. 'The incision is made inside the eye area so there is no visible scarring', emphasises Mr Coghlan. He prefers to carry out lower-eye surgery when his patients are under a general anaesthetic, although he uses a local for those patients who are undergoing upper-eye surgery. Both procedures leave bruising and some swelling for approximately a week.

Liposuction and liposculpture

Liposuction – in which fat is sucked out of the patient's body – can be carried out on various parts of the body, although the thigh area is the most popular. 'The latest technique, called "ultrasonic-assisted liposuction", uses an ultrasound frequency to break down the fatty emulsion before sucking it out,' Mr Coghlan explains. As usually occurs after any loss of weight, the skin has to shrink back, which is why reputable surgeons will only carry out liposuction on patients who have good skin elasticity.

The type of anaesthetic used depends on the size of the area to be treated. Patients need to wear a support garment for four weeks afterwards, followed by regular massage to soften the skin which, incidentally, can take from six weeks to three months. Liposculpture is a less drastic procedure than liposuction: 'We use a fine canulas syringe to remove superficial body fat or inject autologous [the patient's own] fat into hollow areas,' says Mr Coghlan.

Stomach tucks

A flabby tummy can be firmed up with a tummy tuck (abdominoplasty): 'We remove fat and tighten up the skin,' says Mr Coghlan. 'The scar is disguised by the pubic-hair line.' A tummy tuck requires a general anaesthetic and recovery can take several weeks.

HOW TO ACQUIRE A GORGEOUS BODY

Sumptuous skin, shapely legs and a firm, toned body – these sound like the credentials of a supermodel, but achieving them is easier than you think. All it takes is a little discipline and a few tips from the supermodels' own personal trainer.

You may not share Elle Macpherson's vital statistics, but you can still have a desirable body. Before we look at how you can achieve this, let me introduce you to Radu – a fitness guru so famous that he requires no second name. This delightful Romanian opened his Physical Culture Center in New York in 1977 and is now undeniably the most imitated fitness instructor on the planet. By putting Cindy Crawford and a whole host of celebrities, models, dancers and actors through their paces – not to mention getting them to hold a few rather uncompromising positions – Radu has cultivated the bodies of some of the world's most beautiful people. Here he shares his trade secrets with you.

Why bother exercising?

Sit back and be a couch potato if you like, but don't then expect to have a good physique. Exercise is the key to a better body and is paramount when it comes to looking good. With the right training you can resculpt your body: a tighter bottom, firmer thighs, flatter stomach and more shapely legs can all be yours if you get into gear. Start exercising now and you will firm up any problem areas before they get out of hand.

But as Radu stresses, the benefits of exercising surpass aesthetic considerations alone: 'Because in this day and age we lead such sedentary lifestyles, not only are physical activities and sports a health necessity, they are of great importance if we are to obtain balance in our lives', says Radu. 'Exercise is like a very efficient short vacation, which can release stress and give a new perspective on your problems. Physical activities also help you to develop qualities of courage, honesty, discipline, quick decision-making and action-taking.'

Exercise is proven to be a mood enhancer. Because exercising encourages the production of endorphins (the body's natural painkillers) which give you a natural high, after each workout you will feel on top of the world. And, by increasing the blood supply to your brain and stimulating the production of neurotrophins (the brain's growth factor), working out also increases your mental capacity. A fit, strong body means that you will have greater physical reserves that you can draw upon in times of stress and illness.

Convinced of the merits of exercising? If so, before you make a hasty decision as to which exercise is right for you, assess your body by identifying any weak areas that need working on, and then pick the best exercises with which to tackle them, (see Radu's zone specific exercises on page 142.) Always do what you enjoy and vary your exercise so that you don't become bored.

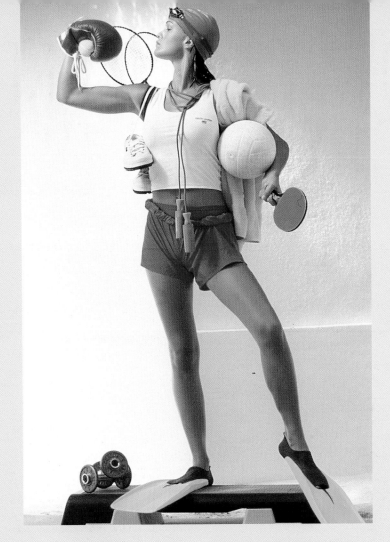

Set yourself a goal

In order to force yourself to switch off the TV and grab your training shoes, you need motivation. To spur you on, imagine how you want to look and keep this image in your head while exercising. Radu suggests that you set yourself some long-term goals like 'I'll change my lifestyle', 'lose weight so that I go down two dress sizes', 'take up squash again' and so on. But no long-term goal can be achieved without also setting short-term targets: 'Say to yourself "I am going to manage three visits to the gym this week or three runs"', insists Radu.

How quickly will you see results?

You *can* alter your body shape, sculpt your bottom and firm up your breasts, but you'll need dedication and patience in order to do so. How intensely you train determines how quickly the results start to show: According to Radu, you will notice a difference after three to four weeks, but the real discoveries are visible after three months. 'Once you see your new physique, nothing will stop you.' If you are starting a new routine go easy to begin with, kicking off with three sessions a week with rest days inbetween and some form of activity at the weekend.

ZONE-SPECIFIC EXERCISES FOR A SEXY, FINELY-HONED BODY

Here Radu has picked a specific exercise for each vital body zone together with lists of the best exercises and sports with which to firm up these areas.

FOR PERT BREASTS

The Exercise: Push-ups

Don't think that you can get away with cissy-style push-ups: if you want great breasts you've got to do the real thing. With your hands and feet on the ground (making sure that they are straight, not turned out), bend your arms a little and do as many press-ups as you can in groups of four. Each day, bend your arms a little more. **Good exercises for the chest:** rope-climbing, all bench-presses, flies, push-ups, dips, pull-overs and exercising with pulleys and elastics. **Good sports for the chest:** wrestling, canoeing, gymnastics, swimming, boxing, throwing sports, pole-vaulting, bench-pressing in power-lifting and rock-climbing.

FOR REFINED BUTT AND THIGHS

The Exercise: Power-skipping

Skip the same way as you did in the playground, jumping higher by adding an explosive push. Do ten skips while standing on each leg, repeat three times. Unlike some exercises, which can make thighs even heavier, skipping keeps them slim. Running with your knees held high, or sprinting so that your feet touch your bottom, are also great ways in which to improve these body zones. **Good exercises for the butt:** skipping, lunges, hip extensions, lateral rotation, abductions, half-squats and reverse hurdles.

Good sports for the butt: track and field sports, speed-running, all jumps, hurdling, fencing, most ball games, gymnastics and swimming. **Good exercises for thighs:** leg extensions, hip flexions, squats (all kinds), leg presses, bench work, rope slalom-jumping, leg rotations and exercising with elastics, pulleys and rubber bands. **Good sports for thighs:** soccer, karate (front-kicking), jumping, track and field sports, cycling, gymnastics (tumbling), ball games, ballet, lifting weights, swimming and sprinting.

FOR FIRMER ABS

The Exercise: Sit-ups

For a truly remarkable, svelte waistline, do several sit-ups with twists. Lie on a mat. Now, with your knees bent towards your right side, bend towards the opposite side. Do as many as you can on each side in groups of four. Another effective exercise is to do lots of twists while standing or sitting, with a broomstick or any other type of stick placed behind your neck. Do three sets for the duration of one minute. The aim of this exercise is not to build rigid abdominal muscles, but to keep this part of your body fluid and supple. **Good exercises for the stomach:** sit-ups, leg lifts, jack-knives, twists, side bends and positions. **Good sports for the stomach:** gymnastics, swimming, boxing, track, field, jumping and running sports.

THE TRAINING PROGRAMME

Physical fitness involves fine-tuning a combination of factors – you may well be able to do the splits but still get out of breath when running for the bus, for example. According to

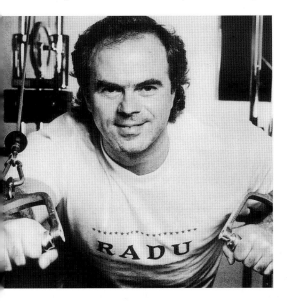

Radu, for optimum fitness you need to address each separate physical quality – strength, speed, endurance, flexibility, balance and co-ordination – in a harmonious way. If that is too much to ask, he suggests following a training programme that includes twenty to thirty minutes of aerobic activity; twenty to thirty minutes of strength training; and five to ten minutes of flexibility exercises. Do this programme at least three times a week.

- **Aerobic exercises:** running, cycling, roller-blading, swimming, canoeing, rowing, basketball, soccer, hiking or walking at a good pace for twenty to thirty minutes will provide you with the necessary aerobic activity for good health and pulmonary function, as well as calorie consumption and fat-burning.
- **Strength and speed training:** do weight-training, gymnastics, boxing, wrestling, callisthenics – push-ups, chin-ups, squats, broad jumps or sit-ups – for twenty to thirty minutes.
- **Flexibility exercises:** doing yoga, ballet or basic stretching exercises for five to eight minutes will provide you with the necessary flexibility to achieve a younger-looking body.

RADU'S TRAINING TIPS

- Three to five sessions of organised physical activities per week are imperative.
- Keep a log of your exercise activity: this will chart your attendance record.
- To give you an indication of the quality of improvement and success of your training, test yourself periodically – once a month, for example – by measuring your body and completing a physical-condition test, for instance, counting how many push-ups, chin-ups or sit-ups you can do.
- Classes are a more dynamic, challenging and efficient way of exercising. You need to arouse your spirit of competition in order to reach the next level of performance.
- Weekend sports activities enable you to test the work that you have been doing during the

week, perhaps by working out at home, outside or at the gym.
- It's great to have a coach or personal trainer who can teach you the proper techniques for practising a sport or performing a complex exercise but, with the exception of special cases, I only recommend a personal trainer to those who lack self-discipline or self-motivation.
- A good body is like an empty shell if it is without substance, so make sure that you eat three meals a day: a hearty breakfast, lunch and a light supper are advisable.
- Between meals, snack on fruit and vegetables: they are the most reliable source of energy yet will not make you put on weight.

THE ROAD TO FITNESS

We all need to be fit on every level – mentally, spiritually and physically.

No one disputes the fact that exercise can work wonders, but keeping fit isn't just about performing near-suicidal aerobics and gruelling sessions on the treadmill. Optimum fitness and well-being rely on the maintenance of mental, emotional and spiritual health, as well as a fit physique. By obtaining an all-round level of fitness you will be empowered to cope with all the challenges that life throws at you.

When we are being bombarded with demands and are suffering from the stresses and stains of life, attaining a state of total well-

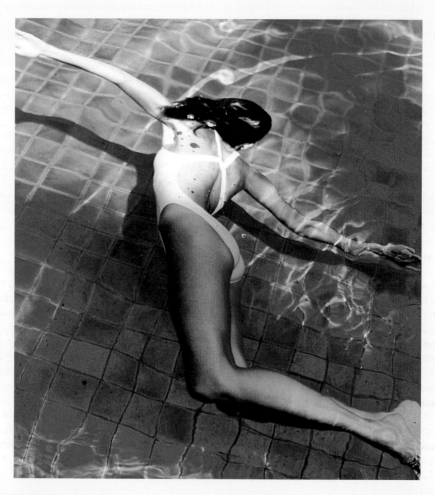

being can seem like a hopeless dream, but if you want to look and feel your best and enjoy life to the full, you'd better start making a few sacrifices. If this means giving up your daily diet of a packet of cigarettes, two bars of chocolate and a bottle of wine, then that's just tough. You may have a zillion and one excuses not to do so, but if you manage to make one or two lifestyle changes you will look and feel so much better. Here are ways to help improve your well-being.

Eliminate Toxins

Toxins are prolific in every aspect of our lives: environmental pollution, cigarette smoke, alcohol, caffeine, drugs, chemicals, pesticides and preservatives contained in processed food all have a toxic effect. An overload of toxins can result in the body's natural detoxifying system becoming sluggish, which can lead to such complaints as cellulite, dull skin, lacklustre hair, allergies, eczema, brittle nails and fatigue.

Detoxifying rids the body of toxins, as well as clearing out any waste products that might be clinging to the colon and preventing the absorbtion of nutrients. In order to avoid toxic build-up, cut down on your intake of alcohol, caffeine and processed foods. Where possible, aim to take natural remedies rather than conventional medicine, and always detoxify your system after a course of antibiotics. Eliminate toxins daily by drinking two litres of water and, every couple of months, cleanse your body for a full day with detoxifying drinks. (Follow the one day home detox on page 150.)

Water power

Water is nature's own internal moisturiser and a great purifier. Drinking plenty of H^2O rehydrates every one of the millions of cells in our body and helps to flush out toxins. Our bodies are made up of seventy-five per cent water. Deprive your body of this essential nectar and you will shrivel up like an old leaf, so aim to drink at least two litres of either mineral or purified water a day. (Unfiltered tap water can, at worst, be contaminated or, in areas where it is safe to drink, can be highly chlorinated, which may destroy nutrients, especially if you're drinking two litres of it.)

Breathe correctly

Oxygen keeps cells healthy and is vital to our looks and well-being. But it's taken the opening of oxygen bars (where people pay for a fix) to highlight its benefits. If you breathe deeply rather than taking shallow gasps, you can absorb plenty of oxygen – absolutely free. This helps oxyginate cells and keeps your complexion fresh looking. In order to check that you are breathing naturally, do the following test: place one hand on your diaphragm and the other on your chest and breathe normally. When you inhale, it should be the hand on your diaphragm that rises higher, not that on your chest. If this isn't happening, concentrate on breathing from your diaphragm and it will soon become second nature.

Meditate

Before you dismiss it as a form of New Age mysticism, let me point out the benefits of meditation: it not only relaxes you, but also clears your mind of trivia. Many people wonder what happens during meditation. The answer is nothing: meditation does not involve thought. However, switching off the mind at will is not easy for most of us, which is why even meditation fanatics need a focus. You can count your breaths, repeat a word (your personal mantra) silently, or emulate a Buddhist monk by chanting. Other ways in which you can focus your mind include staring at an object, such as a candle, a joss stick or even a spot on the wall. If you prefer to close your eyes, you might want to visualise a strong image, such as the face of a loved one, a serene landscape or waves lapping against the shore. Initially, you will need to concentrate hard on your chosen focus in order to avoid your mind becoming side-tracked.

Think positively

A healthy mind is vital to your well-being: if you are not at peace with yourself your biochemistry becomes unbalanced, affecting your looks, self-image and self-confidence. Each day, take time to gather positive thoughts. Positive thinking and an optimistic outlook will keep you both mentally and physically fit. So learn to take the view that your glass of juice is half full – not half empty.

Strive to stay healthy

Boost your body's immune system by eating well and, when necessary, taking a daily multi-vitamin-and-mineral supplement. If you are run-down and in need of a boost, take an immune-system strengthener, such as the herbal supplement echinacea. Regular exercise should protect you against such viruses as colds and flu, while taking cardiospiratory exercise will decrease your risk of developing more major illnesses, such heart disease, diabetes and strokes.

Stop smoking

It's a fact: this dirty habit deprives the skin's cells of oxygen and causes the skin to become thinner, resulting in wrinkles. Dragging endlessly on cigarettes won't only give you ugly, vertical lip lines, but will also affect the skin all over your face and body, not to mention diminishing your pulmonary capacity and increasing the risk of cancer. And as for your breath: if you have, or have had, a partner who smokes, you'll know what I mean by kissing the ashtray!

Follow a fitness plan

Commit yourself to some form of exercise three times a week. Plan ahead and, whether you are swimming, walking or working out in the gym, enter your exercise sessions into your diary and only break them for a justified reason (just because you couldn't be bothered doesn't count).

Swim towards fitness

Swimming is one of the best all-round exercises and, if you swim fast for at least twenty minutes, you will improve your pulmonary capacity and tone up your body. In order to exercise different parts of your body, alternate your stroke. Kicking hard with a float will tone your bottom and legs, while doing the breaststroke will sculpt your shoulders and firm your breasts.

Pirouette yourself fit

Whether you are boogieing until the early hours of the morning, dancing the salsa in a body-hugging clinch with a partner, or doing ballet, contemporary or line-dancing, dancing is an energetic and expressive way to keep fit.

Keep fit the adventurous way

One way in which you can take the boredom out of keeping fit is to get involved in something a little more adventurous than just pumping weights: kickboxing, power-boarding, climbing, aqua-aerobics, snorkelling, paint-balling, canoeing or pole-vaulting, for example. If this list doesn't set your heart racing, how about such hair-raising activities as bridge-swinging, paragliding or Velcro barflying?

Walk in the fresh air

It's free, simple and sociable and, if you walk at a reasonably fast pace you will burn off calories, build up your stamina and stimulate your circulation. A stroll in the countryside or by the sea offers the additional benifits of fresh air, which will oxygenate your cells and energise you. If walking is your chosen form of exercise, skip the treadmill and instead stride briskly through a hilly area or try power-walking for an hour, keeping up the same fast pace (approximately four miles per hour) until the bitter end.

Join a class

Working out with others gives you a real buzz. From spin-cycling to aqua-aerobics, classes are a great way to get- and stay-motivated.

Take up a sport

If the idea of wearing a fancy leotard turns you off, why not take up a sport, such as tennis, golf, squash, soccer, volleyball, or basketball? The team spirit will spur you on. Choose a sport that fits in with your lifestyle and fulfils your personal body goals (see page 142 for Body zone sports).

Practise yoga or t'ai chi

An age-old, Chinese martial art involving slow, fluid movements, t'ai chi is becoming increasingly popular these days. And far from being a New Age fad, yoga, in its various forms – in which you perform a series of postures (*asanas*) – has been on every health club's exercise agenda for years. Both methods increase energy, improve flexibility, counteract stress and tension, and instil a feeling of calm in the mind and body.

A GUIDE TO HOME EXERCISE

By *Zest* magazine's Deputy Editor Sally Brown

Many of us now choose to work out at home rather than at a gym, usually because it saves both time and money. And it is possible to get – and stay – in great shape with home exercise if you approach it as seriously as if you were paying membership fees to a gym. Schedule times for your workouts each week (aim for three to four for best results), put them in your diary and stick to them as you would to other appointments. You may find that exercising in the morning works best because there is less danger of something coming up that causes you to put it off.

One thing that you do miss out on when you work out at home is the professional advice that you get from a good gym. Understanding more about fitness will help you to exercise better, for example, finding out how the muscles in your bottom work will tell you which exercises to do to target them. A good starting point is reading a book, like *Fitness and Health* by Brian J. Sharkey (Human Kinetics, 1996) or Karen Voight's *Precision Training* (Boxtree, 1997). Another option is to invest in a set of personal-training sessions; a good trainer will tailor a programme for you according to how much you can afford.

When it comes to equipment, you don't need to splash out on a stationary cycle or treadmill – unless you know that this is your favourite way of working out and that you will use it regularly. Otherwise, all you need to invest in are a few basics, as follows.

● A good, supportive pair of training shoes to prevent exercise injuries.

● A couple of good exercise videos; interchange them so that you don't get bored and your body doesn't get used to them. Try Karen Voight's 'Streamline Fitness', which includes an aerobic warm-up and exercises for the upper body, legs and bottom, as well as a yogic relaxation session

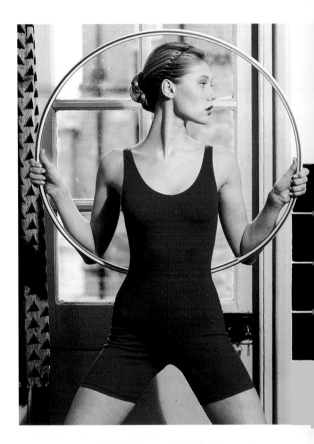

for strength and flexibility, or Marcia Heaner's 'Perfect Curves Workout', a combination of both high- and low-impact aerobics and body-sculpting moves with weights.

● A set of weights to make resistance exercises more effective. Buy a set of both 3lb and 5lb dumbbells (available from department stores and good sports shops). Don't go for ankle weights – if you're doing a leg lift an ankle weight will strain your knee. Instead, hold the dumbbell on your thigh, above your knee.

ENERGY-BOOSTERS

Energy gives us the vitality and stamina that we need to survive if we want to enjoy life to the full. Yet there are many factors that can sap our energy and leave us feeling drained and lethargic, including stress, overwork, menstruation, pollution, changes in the climate, and spending too much time sitting in front of computer and television screens.

If you want to feel bright and breezy there are several ways in which you can boost your energy. Breaking any bad habits and re-evaluating your lifestyle, for example, will sustain your energy levels long term, while as a short-term solution you can send your energy levels soaring upwards with such instant pick-me-ups as energising drinks.

A DOZEN STRATEGIES TO LEAVE YOU EXHILARATED WITH ENERGY

1 Exercise regularly and you will be bursting with energy. When you come home from work you probably feel more like crashing out in front of the TV than rushing off to the health club or going out into the cold for a run but, even then, exercise is guaranteed to revive your energy. However, it's no good spending all of Saturday making up for your lack of activity during the week: unless you exercise regularly – at least three times a week – a sudden surge of exercise could drain your energy. Walk your way to having energy. Even as little as five minutes can help re-energise you.

2 Avoid becoming highly stressed: this saps your energy reserves.

3 Eat breakfast or your energy levels will drop by mid-morning and you will find it more difficult to concentrate. Wholemeal bread, cereal, yoghurt or fruit are less likely to leave you feeling hungry later than white bread or croissants.

4 Cut out caffeine which will help to stabilise any fluctuating blood-sugar levels that might sap your energy. Caffeine, especially in coffee, leaves you feeling depleted of energy after the initial buzz has worn off.

5 Drink two litres of water a day as dehydration can cause fatigue. You will also help to flush out any toxins that might rob you of energy by preventing essential nutrients from being absorbed by the body.

6 Detoxify your body regularly: this will kick-start a sluggish body system.

7 Cut out sugary snacks: for an instant energy boost, hikers and climbers munch their way through bars of Kendal Mint Cake (which is effectively made of pure sugar). Too much of such sticky stuff, however, causes fluctuating blood-sugar levels which, in the long term, can deplete your energy. Nibble energy-packed nuts, raisins, seeds and fruit, instead.

8 Get plenty of sleep: this may seem obvious, but a good night's sleep is one of the best energy-revivers.

9 Eat for energy: energy-giving foods include complex carbohydrates, such as whole grains, vegetables and pulses. Fruit, especially bananas, is also a natural energiser. Supplements that help to boost energy include co-enzyme Q10, vitamin B and the minerals zinc, magnesium, iodine and chromium.

10 Have a positive outlook: your mental attitude can affect your energy levels.

11 Check your health: a health problem may be undermining your energy levels, such as a sluggish liver, food intolerance or candida – a yeast disorder that leaves you feeling lethargic. If you have had a clean health check yet are still lacking in energy, consider such complementary therapies such as naturopathy.

12 Breathe deeply: every deep breath you take delivers oxygen to your cells and energises you.

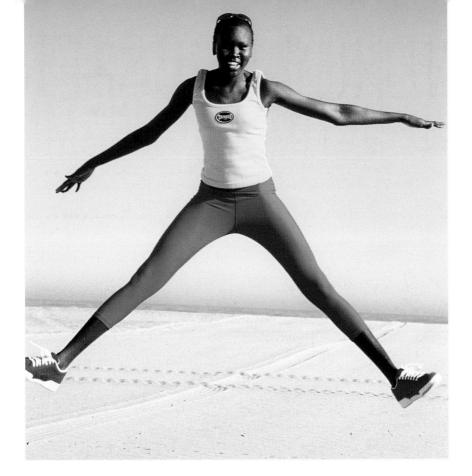

INSTANT ENERGISING PICK-ME-UPS

- **Natural energisers** include guarana, Korean ginseng, aloe-vera juice, kelp, Bioforce's Emergency Essence, co-enzyme Q10 and the Siberian herb *Eleutherococcus senticosus*.
- **Energising drinks:** choose a manufactured healthy nectar that contains such natural stimulants as ginseng and guarana, and boosts energy in a sensible way, like Purdey's or X.TRA. You could also make your own energy-boosting fruit or vegetable drink. Here's a home-made fruit shake for you to try: mix one part pineapple juice to one part skimmed milk with a banana in a blender. Chill it in the fridge before drinking.

- **A cold shower** is an invigorating way in which to refresh and revive yourself instantly. Wimps can start by standing under lukewarm water and then turn the dial towards cold – slowly!
- **Energy-boosting beauty products** include Origins' Sensory Energy Boost On The Spot Gel and Jump Start Body Wash, Virgin Vie's Energy In A Can, Tisserand's Energise and Aveda's Energising Composition Body Oil.
- **Pressing the pericardium-7 acupressure point:** Health and beauty guru Bharti Vyas suggests placing your thumb in the centre of your inner wrist's crease and applying pressure to it by using a pumping action for sixty seconds.

THE ONE-DAY HOME SPA AND DETOX PROGRAMME

If the word 'detoxification' conjures up unappetising images of grapefruit diets, or plastic tubes and having your insides sluiced out with water, think again. This home spa and detox programme will rejuvinate your mind, body and soul the more friendly and fun way.

By pampering yourself with luxurious spa treatments you will restore your looks and rejuvenate your mind and body. Here spa and detox professionals – Christine Ambrose, from the world-famous Dorchester Spa, who has treated the likes of Cindy Crawford and Demi Moore, together with Michael O'Connell, who runs the detoxification course 'Cleansing for Change' – give their tips and guidance to ensure that your home spa and detox programme is as professional as possible. To rid your body of toxins, Michael will help you to detoxify your body from the inside, a crucial factor in the quest for beautiful skin, hair and nails. Treat your detox day as the first day of a new, healthier lifestyle.
(N.B. Do not take part in this programme if you are pregnant, underweight or taking medication.)

SPA PREPERATION

Preparing for the day – Create a peaceful, calming haven by removing all distractions. To turn your home into a sanctuary, Christine suggests playing soothing music and lighting scented candles or a burner filled with essential oils.

Spa attire – You'll need a cosy bathrobe, a pair of slippers, plenty of clean towels, foil, a blanket (electric or thermal if possible), a plastic shower cap or clingfilm, mind-and-spirit books and relaxing tapes (of whale music or sounds of waves lapping on the shore).

PREPARE TO DETOX

Detoxify your body from the inside – Do not drink any tea, coffee or alcohol. Instead, Michael suggests sipping such cleansing herbal teas as fennel, dandelion, lemon or ginger, as well as drinking two litres of mineral or purified water to help to rehydrate your body. Kick off your day with one of the detox drinks listed below. Continue to drink these nectars throughout the day, interspersing them with water and herbal tea. For those who cannot survive the day on detoxifying drinks alone, Michael recommends eating a bowl of vegetable broth (made from organic vegetables) at supper time.

Detox drinks – Michael has devised three cleansing and nourishing drinks, which he prescribes during his 'Cleansing for Change' course. Alternate all three drinks throughout the day, drinking no more than four glasses of each drink. **Drink 1:** Blend a selection of organic vegetables of your choice in a juicer, such as celery, fennel, beetroot, leeks and carrots. **Drink 2:** Mix cider vinegar with a teaspoon of honey – this has an antibacterial effect. **Drink 3:** Mix one or two teaspoons of psyllium husk and half a teaspoon of bentonite clay (found in health-food shops), with one-third of a cup of apple juice and the rest with water. Drink immediately. Like a brush, this helps to scrape off internal plaque and soaks up toxins.

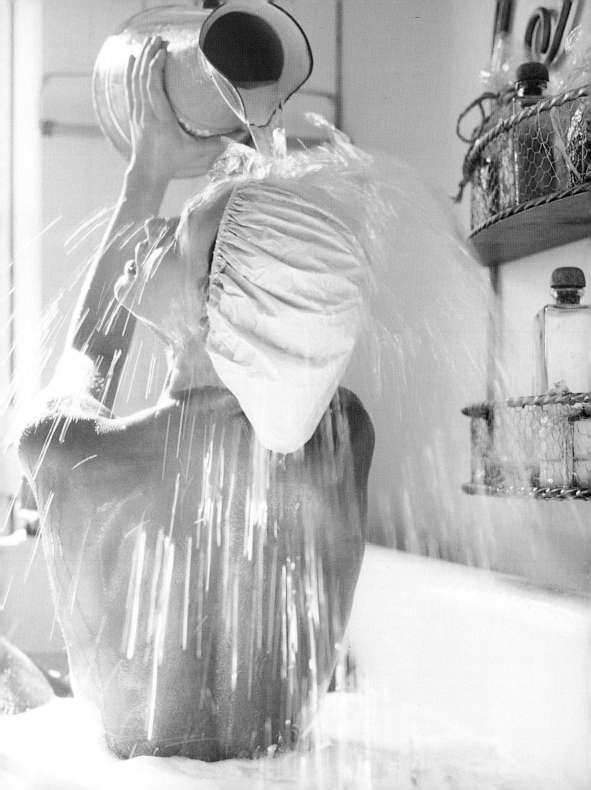

Fruit and Veg detox – If you don't have the ingredients for Michael's drinks, drink freshly prepared juice (made in a juicer), instead. (Ideally, you should stock up on a variety of fruits and vegetables, including carrots, apples, spinach, celery, fennel, leeks and beetroot.) For one of your juice drinks, try the following recipe:

Chiva-Som's beauty-express drink

This nutritious drink was devised by masterchef, Andrew Jacka, of Chiva-Som, one of the world's leading spas.

100g raw spinach, 4 carrots, 2 green apples
600ml water

Wash the vegetables thoroughly (do not peel the apples or carrots). Remove the seeds from the apples and cut them into pieces that will fit into the chute of a vegetable juicer. Pass the apple pieces, spinach and carrots through the juicer. Add water to thin the juice to the desired consistency, and drink.

DETOX AND SPA PROGRAMME

Breath of fresh air – Take half an hour of light exercise outside – such as walking, cycling or gentle jogging – the oxygen that your body takes in will give your skin a healthy glow.

Slow down your pace – To benefit fully from your detoxification day, stop running around like a headless chicken and switch to relaxation mode.

Skin brushing – Take a firm, natural-bristle brush and spend five minutes brushing your body in sweeping movements, working from your toes up to your shoulders; always brush in the direction of your heart. Skin-brushing not only gets the circulation going and sloughs off dead skin, but by cleansing the pores, it eliminates toxins.

Exfoliating shower – Prime your body and prepare your skin in order to make it more receptive to your spa treatments. Christine suggests taking a body scrub or handful of salt into the shower: 'I also find white, granulated sugar works well,' she adds. Exfoliate your body, paying attention to your back, legs, knees, feet and elbows.

Hydrotherapy treatment – Turn your shower into a hydrotherapy jet and give yourself the full spa treatment. 'Direct the shower head towards your body in upward movements, reducing the pressure on sensitive areas,' says Christine, who is a dab hand with the jet. 'This treatment is particularly good for cellulite-prone areas and for releasing tension around the shoulders. Finish off with an invigorating, cold rinse.' For the not so brave, Christine advises acclimatising yourself to the cold water by turning the temperature down gradually. Now rub your body vigorously with a towel, don your bathrobe and slippers, and head for your spa room.

Meditate – Enjoy ten to fifteen minutes of total peace and quiet. Either sit cross-legged in the lotus position or kneel, making sure that your back is straight. Try to keep your mind free of any intrusive thoughts (see page 145 for tips).

Chill out – Spend a decadent hour or so just lounging around in your bathrobe listening to music, reading your mind-and-spirit books or detoxing your mind (see below).

Mind Detox – By relaxing your mind and taking stock of your life you will relax your body, de-stress and see things with more clarity. Sit back in a comfortable chair and, on a notepad, scribble down anything that is playing on your mind (banish all feelings of guilt about work).

• Reassess your lifestyle. Start by writing down ways in which you can change it for the better, for example, by eating more healthily, giving up smoking, cutting down on tea and coffee or joining a gym.

• Look at ways in which you can eliminate stress from your life (see stress-busters on page 170).

• Take steps towards developing a more positive outlook. The idea is to eliminate negative thoughts and improve your view on life by thinking positively.

• Boost your self-esteem. Think of all the positive things about yourself (write a list of them if it helps). Throughout the day, remind yourself that you are gorgeous, special and happy (see page 30 for confidence-boosting tips).

Detoxifying facial – Treat yourself to a luxurious facial. Unless your skin is particularly sensitive or dry, decongest your skin and rid it of impurities by giving yourself a deep-cleansing facial using a mud or clay mask. (Follow the home facial on page 109.)

Eye treat – Rehydrate your under-eye area during your facial by applying a moisturising mask, anti-wrinkle eye pads or cotton-wool pads soaked in milk.

Self body massage – Indulge in a full-body massage using such detoxifying and relaxing oils as E'spa's Restorative Massage Oil or Elemis' De-stress Massage Oil to give your home health spa a professional touch. If you don't possess any aromatherapy oils, a vegetable oil will suffice. (Follow the self body massage on page 173.)

Catnap – Cover your eyes with an eye mask and drift into a deep slumber. If you can't sleep, enjoy the blissful feeling of dosing.

Detoxifying body mask – Smooth on a body mask, such as Borghese's Fango Active Mud Mask, Malki's Dead Sea Mask, The Clay Company's Body Contour Wrap or, simply fuller's earth, which you mix into a paste by adding a little water (this is available from most pharmacies). For best results, Christine advises wrapping yourself in foil before covering your body with prewarmed towels or, better still, an electric or thermal blanket: 'The key is to keep your body as warm as possible,' she says. Leave it on for twenty minutes and then shower it off.

Relaxation and deep-breathing technique – During the twenty minutes you are lying embalmed in your body mask, follow the self relaxation and deep-breathing technique on page 169.

Hair treatment – Put shine, body and bounce back into your hair by applying a rich, nourishing hair treatment or mask of your choice. Pop on a plastic shower cap, wrap your head in foil and then cover with a towel which has been prewarmed. Leave it on for twenty minutes while in your thalassotherapy bath (see below). Sluice off the mask and then treat your hair to a final rinse with purified or mineral water.

Thalassotherapy bath – This is a heavenly spa treatment for the mind and body. To turn your bath into a spa bath, Christine suggests adding a blended aromatherapy oil to the bath water, together with either algae, seaweed or mud. Choose from such products as Thalgo's Thalassobath, E'spa's Detoxifying Seaweed Bath, Boot's Spa Detoxifying Bath, Algascience's Relaxing Bath, or else simply use fresh seaweed from either the sea (if you live close by) or your local supermarket. Mix them into the water (don't run under the tap), light a scented candle, make a headrest by folding up a small towel, and then submerge yourself in the water and soak for at least twenty minutes. After your bath, smooth on a body lotion.

Air bath – Enjoy a feeling of freedom by walking around your home wearing nothing but your birthday suit.

Go to bed early – By the end of the day you'll be feeling totally relaxed, nicely tired and possibly a little light-headed, too, (don't worry about this, it's just your body's reaction to not having been bombarded with all the usual stimulants). To benefit fully from your spa and detox day, don't make any plans for the evening. Put a couple of drops of lavender essential oil onto your pillow and sleep peacefully, knowing that tomorrow you will look and feel like a new person.

A GUIDE TO COMPLEMENTARY
THERAPIES

No longer pigeonholed as 'alternative', holistic therapies and Eastern healing methods have gained credence by treating the cause rather than just the symptoms of a whole range of health and beauty problems, from spotty skin to poor posture.

Acupressure works according to the same principles as acupuncture but uses finger pressure rather than needles to stimulate the acupoints. Having located the main pressure points on your body (with the help of a therapist or good book), you can treat yourself by applying pressure to these points.

Acupuncture is an age-old Chinese therapy that concentrates on the twelve meridians or energy channels which, according to Chinese philosophy, circulate our body and correspond with various body organs. The therapist inserts fine needles into the key pressure points, unblocking the meridians and encouraging the release of *chi*, the body's energy flow. It can treat such beauty problems as acne, and can alleviate dark, under-eye shadows that could be due to a sluggish liver or sinus problems.

Ayurveda treats patients using herbal remedies, oils, massage and detoxifying regimes. This ancient Indian healing system is based on three biological forces or energies, called *doshas*, together with the five elements: earth, water, fire, air and space. By restoring the doshic balance – the body's energy – it can successfully treat skin conditions and other beauty problems.

Colonic irrigation During this procedure, the colon is flushed out with water, which both cleanses it and frees any toxic waste that might be clinging to its walls and preventing the absorption of nutrients. It is regarded as being good for skin problems and general well-being.

Cranial osteopathy This is a gentle form of osteopathy that does not involve any bone-crunching manipulation. By working on the neck and head to release tension and realign the spine, cranial osteopathy is a great antidote to stress and also helps to unblock sinuses, thus ameliorating under-eye shadows.

Herbalism Herbal medicine treats many ailments as effectively as conventional drugs, but without their side effects. For example, echinacea has become a 'wonder' herb for boosting the immune system and fighting such skin conditions as acne, while St John's Wort is lauded as the herbal equivalent of the anti-depressant Prozac. You have the option to visit a herbalist, or purchase herbal preperations, such as echinacea, from health stores or pharmacies.

Homeopathy Therapists believe that many superficial health and beauty problems are caused by underlying disorders, so homeopathic diagnosis involves investigating the patient's lifestyle and medical history. Based on the same principle as inoculation (treating like with like), minuscule amounts of homeopathic substances are used to help treat a barrage of problems, from skin complaints to overcoming blushing.

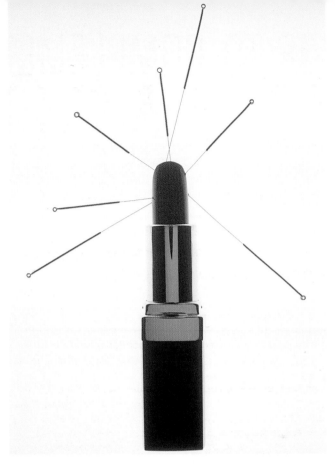

Hypnotherapy Let me assure you that hypnotherapy is not an entertainment-style hypnotic technique in which you are put into a trance at the click of a finger and told to respond to ridiculous demands. Hypnotherapy simply puts you in a state of deep relaxation, which naturally alters your awareness to the level into which we all drift several times a day. Hypnotherapy can help to break bad habits, particularly smoking and binging.

Naturopathy Using a combination of diet, fresh air, water and relaxation, naturopaths believe in the power of nature to heal. Some therapists also practice homeopathy, herbalism and osteopathy, along with their naturopathic treatments. The elimination of toxins plays an important part in naturopathy: practitioners may, for instance, suggest a fast or a wholefood, vegetarian diet.

Osteopathy Working on the body's skeletal framework, osteopaths manipulate the spine and joints to realign bones, muscles and ligaments. Osteopathy is considered good for treating backache, migraine and neck problems, which are often a result of injury or bad posture.

Reflexology Certain points on the feet correspond to the body's major organs and, by using thumb pressure on these points and discovering tender spots, practitioners can diagnose any problems. To help alleviate the disorder, therapists use acupressure and massage on the corresponding points.

Reiki An ancient form of Tibetan healing that is best described as the 'laying-on of hands', in which energy is channelled through the hands of the healer to the patient. The healing works on all levels – physical, emotional, mental and spiritual.

AROMATHERAPY

Succumb to the beautifying and health-giving properties of plant oils.

Aromatherapy was first used as far back as 3000 BC by the Egyptians, who discovered its uses for culinary and therapeutic purposes, as well as in perfumed oils and incense. Natural aromatic essences are extracted from different parts of both wild and cultivated plants, including their flowers, leaves, fruits, seeds, bark and stems, and are then made up into essential oils.

A key ingredient in perfume and in many of the leading skin- and bodycare ranges, essential oils have a wide variety of uses, not just on account of their aroma, but also for their beautifying and therapeutic properties.

Essential oils are sold either in their pure form or blended with such carrier oils as almond, wheatgerm or jojoba. Reassuringly, there are now many specialist companies that provide safe and effective pure oils and blends. Dilute essential oils with a carrier oil for massage, sprinkle blended oils into a bath, or add a few drops to body lotions or natural ingredients to make your own range of beauty preparations (see page 164 for DIY recipes).

One of the leading authorities on aromatherapy is Susan Harmsworth, head of E'spa, which manufactures a range of beauty, spa and bath products based on aromatherapy. Susan has seen how more and more people are turning to aromatherapy for both health and beauty remedies. Aromatherapy is, for example, now widely used in conjunction with massage to help relax the body. 'As we enter the new millennium with our man-made stress, many of us are seeking home remedies and are relying on soothing baths, refreshing aromas and the healing hands of a qualified aromatherapist,' explains Susan. 'As always, nature has never let us down. Let's hope that humankind realises the precious gifts of aromatherapy for its own sake!'

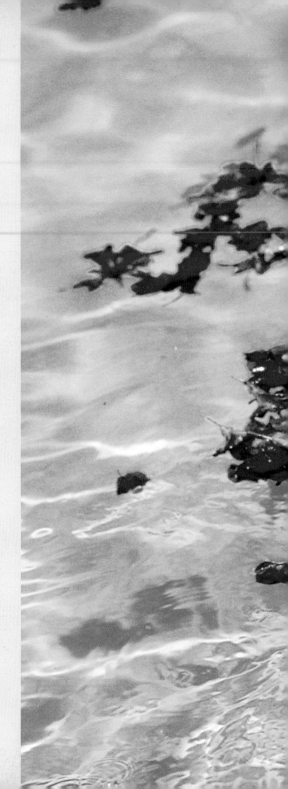

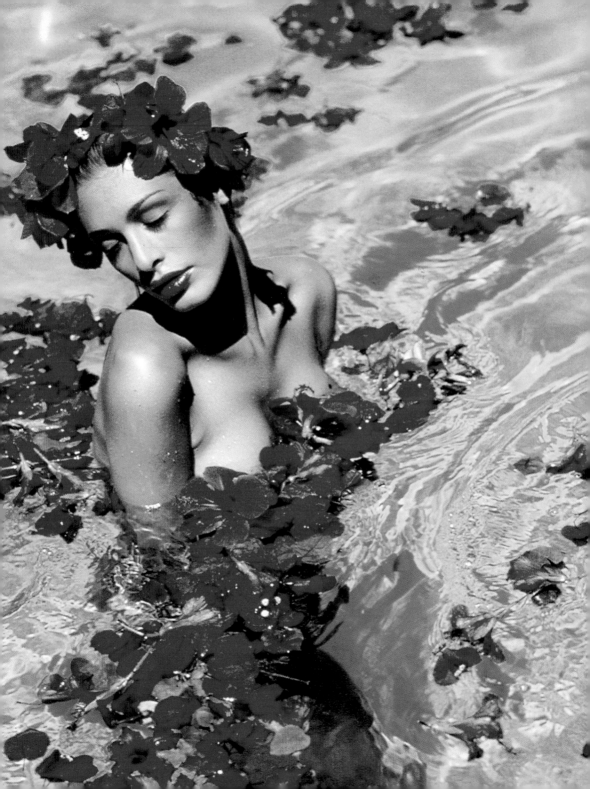

TREATING BEAUTY PROBLEMS WITH AROMATHERAPY

If you are using essential oils rather than blended oils, having purchased the purest essential oil that you can find, you will need to blend it with what is termed a 'base' or 'carrier' oil. When the application is to be used on your face, walnut, wheatgerm or avocado oils make good base oils, whereas you can use any vegetable oil you like for your body. Mix two to three drops of essential oil to every 10ml of base oil. You don't have to stick to one essential oil: for example, for cellulite you could blend juniper, cypress and lemon essential oils with your base oil. Here is a list of common beauty ailments and the most suitable oils with which to treat them:

- **Acne:** tea-tree, calendula, camomile, mint, neroli, patchouli, thyme or lavender essential oil. Mix essential oil with a base oil of jojoba.
- **Bad circulation:** neroli, lemon, rose or cypress essential oil. Use a base oil of your choice.
- **Blackheads:** juniper or neroli essential oil added to a base oil of jojoba.

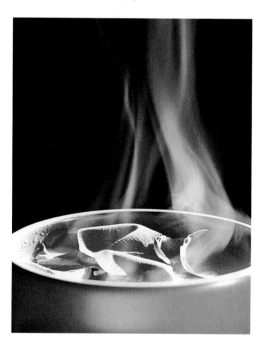

- **Broken capillaries:** cypress, rose or calendula essential oil added to a base oil of avocado.
- **Cellulite:** juniper, cypress, lemon or rosemary essential oil added to a base oil of wheatgerm.
- **Dandruff:** tea-tree, rosemary, cedarwood, patchouli, thyme or bay essential oil. Use grape-seed as the base oil.
- **Dry skin and wrinkles:** rose, benzoin, galbanum, rosemary, myrrh, frankincense, jasmine or lavender essential oil. Add to a base oil of avocado, wheatgerm or walnut.
- **Eczema and dermatitis:** cedarwood, calendula, frankincense or camomile essential oil in a base oil of avocado or wheatgerm.
- **Sunburn:** lavender or camomile essential oil in a base oil of wheatgerm.
- **Weak nails:** frankincense or myrrh essential oil in a base oil of almond.

AROMATHERAPY PLUS

Go into sensory overload by bringing aromatherapy into your life in many different ways. Sprinkle your favourite essential oil on a burner, light an aromatherapy candle or attach a light-bulb ring containing an essential oil to a lamp. Incense sticks, potpourri and scented pebbles will also bring wonderful aromas into your home. Alternatively, drench some cotton-wool balls in your favourite essential oil and pop them into a discreet corner of a room.

AROMATHERAPY PROPERTIES

Essential oils yield different effects on the mind, body and soul. Here is a list of property-inducing essential oils:

- **Uplifting:** jasmine, basil and lemon grass.
- **Stimulating:** juniper, rosemary, mint, lavender, marjoram, eucalyptus, bergamot and rose.
- **Healing/antiseptic:** tea-tree, lavender, eucalyptus, clove, camphor and pine.
- **Detoxifying:** lemon and juniper.
- **Balancing:** geranium and patchouli.
- **Relaxing, calming and soothing:** ylang-ylang, clary sage, pine, sandalwood, neroli, geranium, lavender, camomile, jasmine, benzoin, patchouli and frankincense.

A GUIDE TO AROMATHERAPY

by E'spa's Susan Harmsworth

Essential oils are derived from aromatic plants. They are highly volatile substances, with varying degrees of evaporation. How and where the plant is picked is vital to the pure energy and therapeutic properties of the pure essential oil. Many manufactures adulterate the oils, mixing plant species or supplementing with synthetic material, so impairing the holistic balance of the oil. It is therefore imperative that when purchasing oils the species, source, history and a full listing of benefits are known. Organically grown plants are not contaminated by chemical pesticides, which are difficult to remove in the distillation process. When selecting essential oils, these are the general points for you to consider:

1 Know the difference between a pure essential oil, a blended aromatic type and one of synthetic origin. Pure aroma oils are normally packaged in small, darkened-glass bottles as ultraviolet light destroys their fine, delicate fragrance. Look for the species and history of the oil, as well as the supplier's accreditation.

2 All oil packaging should carry the date of manufacture and the life span of the oil, with cautions and warnings clearly marked.

3 Always seek professional advice before using essential oils; remember that in their undiluted form they may be toxic and may cause nasty side effects. A qualified aromatherapist will be registered and will be able to provide you with recognised, certified qualifications.

4 Essential oils should be diluted in a vegetable-based carrier oil for massage (two to three drops in 10ml of such base oils as almond, grape-seed or jojoba will give a one per cent blend).

5 When pregnant or nursing, many precautions are needed, and the use of essential oils is not recommended unless they have been selected by a qualified practitioner.

6 Warm, aromatic baths taken by candlelight are an effective and healthy way in which to remove the trauma and stress of everyday life. Many companies, including E'spa, preblend essential oils with a natural dispersant so that the oils diffuse into the water, giving softness to the skin, and balance and harmony to the mind, without leaving an oily residue around the bath.

7 Diffusing oils in burners, aroma stones and light-bulb rings can change the energy in a room, ridding it of unpleasant odours and sterilising a sick room.

8 Only in an emergency situation, such as when treating an insect sting or bite, may lavender or tea-tree oil be used in an undiluted form on the skin as all oils are dermacaustic in varying degrees.

9 The natural components of aromatic oils are compatible with the intricate and delicate balance of our bodies, making their advantages over conventional medicine considerable. But more is not necessarily better, and bear in mind that oils remain in the body for anything from one hour to several weeks after application. So the most important factor to remember when using oils is that too much and only a little knowledge can be dangerous.

10 Before using essential oils, always check with your doctor if you are taking drugs, are post-operative or are under medical supervision. Store oils in a cool, dark place and keep them out of the reach of children.

FRAGRANCE

Fragrance has a magical, mystical power: a mere whiff of perfume has
driven men crazy with passion and has seduced women into falling madly in love. Fragrance
can also lift your spirits and calm your mind.

Marilyn Monroe claimed that Chanel No 5 was the only thing that she wore in bed; she may have been nude, but without her scent she would have been stark naked. Fragrance is *de rigueur* for the modern woman, for not only does it add the finishing touch to your image, but it is also your personal signature and your stamp of identity. Floral and fresh, woody and seductive, oriental and citrusy, there are many wonderful formulations available from the different fragrance families to suit every character, mood and moment. Aim to build up your very own wardrobe of fragrances, while appointing your overall favourite as your signature scent.

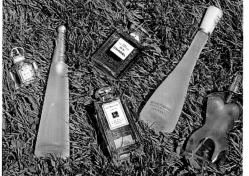

Scent isn't exclusive to perfume, bath and shower products or body lotions: you can bring fragrance into your home with scented candles, aroma pebbles, potpourri, incense sticks and room mists. There's even a linen scent available to give your sheets that freshly-washed, line-dried smell, as well as diet scents – patches that you stick on your body and sniff when you feel hungry to help stave off any food cravings.

Because smells transmit along the olfactory nerve to the brain's memory centre, fragrance can instantly evoke memories and stir up emotions, which is why we often associate a perfume with a particular person or place. Scent has the power to manipulate your mood. Scientific studies have discovered that stimulating the brain through perfume can awaken the senses, reduce stress and anxiety, ease depression, alleviate fatigue and have an uplifting effect. Fragrance houses were quick to launch calm-inducing scents that enhance both physical and mental well-being, but don't think that you have to douse yourself in it – it only takes a tiny amount for olfactory stimulation of the brain to occur.

You may have noticed how the smell of your perfume alters throughout the day. These different levels of smell – which take place in three stages – are termed 'notes'. Not unlike a piece of music, they kick off with the heady rush – caused by the 'top' notes – that hit you when you first spray or dab on a fragrance. After a few minutes of exposure to oxygen, the top notes give way to more subtle, 'heart' notes. These gradually develop into the underlying, 'base' notes, which unfold and linger throughout the fragrance song.

FRAGRANT FACTS

- Scent is sold in different forms, which are determined by strength. The most concentrated is *parfum*, followed by *eau de parfum, parfum de toilette, eau de toilette, eau de cologne* and *eau de fraîche*.
- Keep the bottle away from direct sunlight and heat, and help to prolong the life of your scent by storing it in its box.
- A fragrance reaches its 'best-by' date after a year/year and a half, so unless you wear the same scent every day and are likely to use it up, you'd be better off buying a small bottle.
- Rather than carrying your perfume bottle in your handbag, decant a small amount into an atomiser. Not only will this lighten your load, but the bulk of your perfume won't be exposed to varying degrees in temperatures.
- As perfume reacts badly to heat and can cause allergic reactions, don't wear any while sunbathing (unless it is a sun-proof formulation).

A woman who doesn't wear perfume has no future.
    Coco Chanel (1883–1971).

FRAGRANCE LAYERING

Jo Malone developed her own fragrance range a decade ago, which now has a cult following among celebrities and models. An instrumental figure in the revival of fragrance layering (also known as combining), Jo believes that the beauty of it is that it allows you to become a perfumer and create a scent that is unique to you.

Fragrance takes many different shapes and forms, and a number of perfume houses offer a selection of fragranced products within their ranges, including body lotion, bath oil, shower gel, soap, deodorant, shampoo and conditioner. Most of us would assume that the ultimate luxury would be to layer products from the same fragrance range, but according to Jo this could be overdoing it. 'By combining a shower gel from one fragrance and a perfume from another, you can create your very own scent. For example: follow a grapefruit body lotion with a tuberose cologne. You may want to stick to the same family of fragrances, such as floral, or be really bold and wear more than one actual perfume,' says Jo, who rarely leaves the house without spraying on at least two.

A GUIDE TO CHOOSING A FRAGRANCE

by Guerlain's professeur des parfums, Roja Dove
The undisputed fragrance guru shares his expertise to help you find a scent that will suit your lifestyle, character and moods.

- Fragrance is a very individual and subjective thing, so when shopping for perfume my advice is always to go alone.
- Never test a fragrance if you are already wearing one.
- You may have several fragrances that you like, but allocate one as your signature fragrance. Don't worry about smelling like all the other thousands of consumers who have bought the same brand: if you've purchased a good-quality fragrance that contains natural raw materials, the perfume will not smell identical on any two people. At Guerlain we have a saying: 'It's the woman who perfumes our perfumes, not the perfume who perfumes the woman'.
- Spray the tester all over you, leave the shop and live with it for a day. Remember, a fragrance takes four to six hours to develop, and it's the base notes that you will have to live with. A perfume is like a lover – you never know what it is like until you've slept with it!
- The consumers of sixty per cent of all fragrances sold have been influenced by the brand name or advertising. However, the right fragrance should be chosen not by your conscious mind, but by your subconscious and what the smell conjures up in your imagination.
- Fragrances come in different families, such as floral and oriental. Try a scent from each family rather than picking one that you think is right for a particular season or occasion.

TURN TO NATURE

In this high-tech age many of us are reverting to nature and choosing an organic beauty elixir. But rather than shunning science in favour of all things natural, we can enjoy the benefits of both.

Peek into any model or celebrity's beauty kit and you'll be sure to find an abundance of natural-based products from ranges manufactured by Aveda, Dr Hauschka, Elemis, Blackmore, Nuxe, Jurlique, E'spa, Harper, Kiehl's, Origins and Philosophy, to name but a few.

While the Avedas and Philosophys of this world realised the demand for organic products and bottled them, beauty shops like Lush started dishing up delicatessen-style tubs of 'fresh' face cream made from bananas, strawberries and many other ingredients good enough to eat. This desire for purity isn't just a passing trend, however: The Body Shop has been successfully churning out cucumber water and oatmeal scrubs since 1976 while, since 1851, Kiehl's has been concocting the kind of natural potions that no model today would be without.

A large percentage of the products that we slap onto our faces and bodies are ingested by the skin and absorbed into the blood stream, which is one of the reasons why organic skincare products are in demand. Extending much further than skincare alone, these natural-based ranges – made from plants, flowers, herbs, spices, marine algae, fruit and vegetables – often encompass make-up, hair-, sun- and bodycare preparations and, even babycare and household products.

With the mainstream cosmetics giants shaking off their clinical image and tapping into nature by using more plant extracts, marine vegetation and minerals of the land, they – and we – could arguably be said to be shunning science for nature. But as the head of Estée Lauder, William P. Lauder, explains, rather than opting for one or the other, companies like Origins, for example, have cleverly married science with centuries-old remedies to give the consumer the best of both worlds.

Before you rush out and buy decanter-sized flacons of 'natural' products, don't be misled into thinking that their ingredients are always a hundred per cent natural. With the exception of one or two ranges, most contain tiny amounts of synthetic substances, such as preservatives, emulsifiers and carrying agents. These are necessary – especially when used in conjunction with other, more unstable ingredients – to allow the products to be kept and used for longer than just a few weeks. In the better ranges, synthetic ingredients only make up a tiny percentage of the product and are fairly innocuous. It's also worth remembering that not only are some plant-derived products toxic, but that all plants rely on chemical reactions caused by sunlight and soil for survival, so even 'natural' isn't necessarily a hundred per cent 'pure'.

Some companies, however, are jumping on the 'natural' bandwagon with products that only contain minute traces (as little as one per cent) of authentically natural ingredients. This is now changing as, in the USA, packaging has to carry a list of all the product's entire ingredients. In order to play it safe, you should only buy products from better-known manufacturers – such as Aveda, Jurlique and all the others listed at the beginning of this section – that are acknowledged as containing the highest possible amount of natural ingredients.

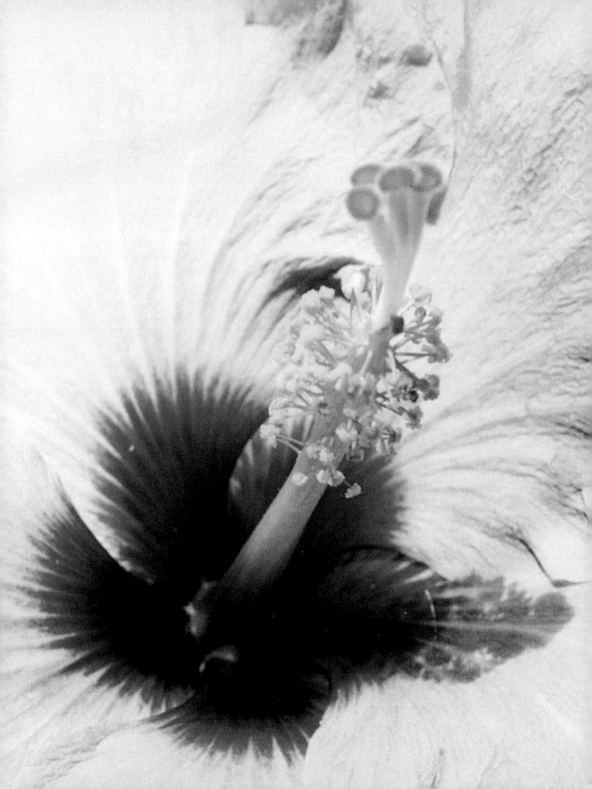

DO IT YOURSELF:
HOME-MADE BEAUTY RECIPES

Home-made preparations are both cheap and fun to make, so start
raiding your kitchen cupboards for DIY beauty solutions.

YOUR BEAUTY LARDER

Stock up on the ingredients you need to make the beauty recipe of your choice.

- **Foods:** avocados, honey, papaya, fine oatmeal, ground almonds, finely-ground sea salt, cucumber, banana, eggs and natural yoghurt.
- **Liquids:** witch hazel, glycerine, rose-water, elderflower water and cider vinegar.
- **Powders:** kaolin or white clay, fuller's earth, crushable vitamin-C tablets or vitamin-C powder, powdered kelp, turmeric spice and borax.
- **Oils:** almond, wheatgerm, walnut, avocado and jojoba.
- **Solids:** beeswax and coconut oil.
- **Essential oils:** tea-tree, rose and geranium.
- **Tools:** a piece of muslin, a saucepan, blender, teaspoon, dessertspoon, woodenspoon, whisk, an old make-up brush and cotton gloves.

N.B. The above ingredients can be found in most supermarkets, pharmacies or health food stores.

BEAUTY RECIPES

Deep-cleansing mud mask
1 dessertspoon fuller's earth
2 teaspoons cider vinegar
Mix the ingredients into a paste and apply it to your face immediately. Wait until the mask has hardened before washing it off.

Revitalising clay mask
2 dessertspoons clay or kaolin
¼ cucumber
Peel the cucumber and blend it into pulp. Remove most of the liquid, saving a little to mix with the powder to make a paste. (Keep the remainder of the liquid to make a cucumber freshener by adding a little witch hazel.) Now add the pulp, apply it to your face and leave it on for ten minutes.

Seaweed conditioning mask
2 dessertspoons powdered kelp
1 dessertspoon glycerine
1 dessertspoon rose-water
Mix the ingredients into a paste. Apply it to your face and leave it on for ten minutes.

Skin-firming enzyme mask
1 papaya, peeled
1 egg white
1 teaspoon honey
Whisk the egg white. Now mash the peeled papaya with a fork and mix it with the honey. Apply it to your face and leave it on for twenty minutes.

Wrinkle-smoothing mask
1 teaspoon wheatgerm oil
1 vitamin-C tablet, crushed, or 1 teaspoon vitamin-C powder
Muslin cloth
Cut the muslin into a mask shape by making holes for your eyes and lips. Mix the vitamin-C powder with the oil. Put the muslin mask on your face and then brush on the paste. Leave it on for twenty minutes, then peel off the cloth and rinse your face with lukewarm water.

Nourishing mask
1 avocado
1 teaspoon honey
Mash the avocado and mix it with the honey. Spread the paste onto your face and leave it on for ten minutes.

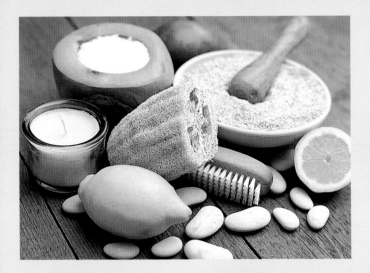

meantime, dissolve the borax powder in the boiling water and add it to the pan, along with the almond and geranium oil, stirring vigorously. Remove it from the heat and immediately whisk the mixture (using an electric or hand whisk), until it resembles a smooth paste. Decant into a jar for future use.

Gentle toner
Rose-water
Elderflower water
Mix one part rose-water with one part elderflower water and decant the liquid into a bottle. If your skin is oily, substitute the elderflower with witch hazel.

All-round nourishing cream
3 teaspoons beeswax
6 dessertspoons wheatgerm oil
3 dessertspoons boiling water
6 drops rose oil
1½ teaspoons borax
Melt the beeswax in a saucepan over a moderate heat. In the meantime, dissolve the borax powder in the boiling water and add it to the pan, along with the wheatgerm and rose oil, stirring vigorously. Remove it from the heat and immediately whisk the mixture (using an electric or hand whisk), until it resembles a smooth paste. Decant it into a jar for future use.

Nourishing hair mask
1 dessertspoon almond oil
1 egg yolk
1 banana, mashed
Mix the oil with the egg yolk and banana, then apply the paste to your hair. Leave it on for twenty minutes.

Eastern-promise tanning mask
1 teaspoon turmeric spice
1 dessertspoon natural yoghurt
Mix the turmeric with the yoghurt. Apply the paste to your face and leave it on for ten minutes. This mask gives a slight tanning effect to the skin.

Restorative hand and nail treat
Wheatgerm or almond oil
Cotton gloves
Warm a little of the oil in a pan. Massage it into your hands and nails and then put on cotton gloves (heat the gloves on a radiator first). Leave them on for an hour or overnight, if possible.

Gentle face scrub
1 dessertspoon fine oatmeal
1 teaspoon avocado or walnut oil for dry skin, or jojoba oil for oily skin
Mix the oatmeal and oil together, then apply the scrub to a wet face, using circular movements.

Anti-blemish back scrub
1 dessertspoon finely ground sea salt
2 drops tea-tree oil
1 teaspoon glycerine
Add the tea-tree oil to the glycerine and then mix in the salt. Take the paste into the shower and scrub your back.

Moisturising all-over exfoliant
1 dessertspoon ground almonds
1 teaspoon honey
Mix the honey and ground almonds together and then use the scrub in the shower or while washing your face.

Balancing cleanser
3 teaspoons beeswax
6 dessertspoons almond oil
3 dessertspoons boiling water
3 teaspoons coconut oil
1½ teaspoons borax
6 drops geranium oil
Melt the beeswax and coconut oil in a saucepan over a moderate heat. In the

PERFECT POSTURE

Having good posture instantly makes you appear more confident, inches taller and far more attractive. While the furthest slouching will get you is to the auditions for *The Hunchback of Notre Dame.*

Unless having a concave chest, Quasimodo hunched back and a chin angled like Concorde sounds attractive to you, then I suggest that you refrain from slouching or rounding your shoulders. For starters, poor posture is detrimental to your looks, while a good stance imparts both extra inches and self-confidence. Here are a few words of wisdom that were recounted to me by my osteopath, which have stuck since my teens: 'If an unattractive woman holds herself well, regardless of her lack of good looks, she will appear more beautiful than the gorgeous woman who slouches.'

Bad deportment not only damages the spine but can also affect your general health, leading to back problems, headaches, poor circulation and indigestion. If you are hunched over, it is also unlikely that you are breathing correctly, so you are thus depriving your body of oxygen. What's even more frightening is that continual slouching could permanantly alter your body shape.

You can discipline yourself to walk tall, but it takes a little more commitment than just sticking your shoulders back and your chest out. In the 1950s and 1960s, models used to balance books on their heads while practising their walk – you may giggle at the thought, but there's still something to be said for this traditional method of deportment. Regular exercise – in particular those exercises which strengthen the abdominal and back muscles – will help you to hold yourself straighter. Be aware of your stance wherever you are, be it in the supermarket, at a party – and especially – at home, as this is where you are most likely to revert to any bad habits.

POSTURE-IMPROVING TECHNIQUES

- **Self-help exercise:** stand up straight and imagine that you have a piece of string attached to your chest that is lifting you towards the ceiling. While raising your chest, hold your stomach in and tuck in your bottom; refrain from tilting your pelvis. Now make sure that your chin is positioned correctly and that your shoulders are neither hunched up nor forced back, just relaxed.
- **The Alexander Technique:** having discovered a connection between the mind, emotions and posture, actor Frederick Alexander devised the technique over a century ago. Often practiced on a one-to-one basis, The Alexander Technique involves a therapist teaching you a series of gentle exercises with which to retrain your posture, working in particular on the neck area.
- **Pilates:** this excellent form of body-conditioning was pioneered by gymnast Joseph Pilates. By using certain movements, Pilates works on strengthening weak muscles (in particular the abdominals) and ultimately retrains you to stand well.
- **The Feldenkrais Method:** the brainchild of Moshe Feldenkrais, this method uses a series of floor exercises and manipulation (on a one-to-one basis) to correct bad posture.
- **Yoga and t'ai chi:** either of these, when practised regularly over time, will help you to improve your stance and balance, and regain your natural poise.
- **Rolfing:** through massage therapists realign the body.

BEAUTY SLUMBER

Supermodels swear by it and babies do it all
the time. Sleep is the ultimate beauty treatment – and it's free!

While you are deep in the land of Nod, your skin renews itself at a level untouched by even the most technologically advanced 'miracle' cream. Skin cells reproduce themselves at a faster rate and collagen production speeds up, which explains why, after a restful night's sleep, you wake up looking radiant and feeling energised.

Lack of zzzs will also affect your looks: we've all experienced that morning-after feeling when a nocturnal-looking creature with dark-rimmed eyes and a drab, greyish-looking complexion stares out at us from the mirror. Looks aside, sleep deprivation inhibits your co-ordination and control over situations, lowers the effectiveness of your immune system, leaves you feeling lethargic and tetchy, and heightens your emotions – you will, no doubt, recognise that wretched feeling when you could burst into tears or let rip with rage at the slightest thing. So if the last time you had a proper night's sleep was when your mother tucked you up and read you a bedtime story, make a concerted effort to get more of nature's beautifier.

TIPS FOR PEACEFUL SLUMBER

- **Beautify yourself:** pep up your looks while you sleep by applying treatments to parts of the body that need a particular boost. Apply a face or hair mask, for example, and massage your hands and feet with cream or oil before popping on pre-warmed cotton gloves and socks.
- **How long?** On average, adults need between six-and-a-half and eight hours' sleep, but as the number of hours depends very much on the individual, you should work out your own optimum quota.

- **Clear your mind:** if you've been working late, it is important to unwind before going to bed. Try reading: even if you are wide awake, after a few pages your eyes will tire and you will feel sleepy. Reading also helps to divert your mind from any worries or intrusive thoughts that could otherwise prevent you from sleeping.
- **Relax in a warm bath:** sprinkle your bath water with such sleep-inducing products as Origins' Sensory Therapy Sleep-time Bath Oil, or a bath oil containing lavender or sandalwood.
- **Prepare your boudoir:** make sure that your curtains keep out the light and check that your bed and pillows are comfortable. If you are a light sleeper, muffle any extraneous noise with earplugs for an uninterrupted night's sleep.
- **Insomnia:** if you suffer from sleepless nights, avoid taking sleeping tablets – they may induce sleep but scientists have proved that the quality of sleep is dramatically reduced. Instead, try natural herbal remedies, such as valerian root and passiflora, or sprinkle your pillow with a drop of lavender essential oil.
- **Catching up:** if you've gone to bed with the dawn chorus, don't worry about trying to catch up on every single hour you've lost – your body naturally compensates for missed sleep on the following night by sending you into a deeper, less interrupted slumber. Retiring to bed early for a couple of nights is one of the best ways in which to get back on the sleep track.
- **Bedtime nectar:** avoid drinking coffee before you go to bed – the caffeine will make you more alert. Instead, have a natural, sedative drink, such as camomile, primrose, veberna, lemon-balm tea or hot milk, which contains the amino acid tryptophan and has a sleep-inducing effect.

RELAX AND UNWIND

The phone's ringing, someone's yelling –
it's pandemonium. If you need an antidote to today's stressful living, read on.

What does the word 'relaxation' conjure up in your mind? Sipping ice-cold martini cocktails on a sun-drenched beach, meditating in the lotus position, burying your head in a good book, having an aromatherapy massage or gazing aimlessly at the clouds? The Hale Clinic's Dr Robert D. Russell, a personal-development and stress-management counsellor, points out that relaxation isn't just about lying on a beach or crystal-gazing: 'Relaxation is a combination of three things,' explains Dr Russell. 'You need to balance work with a mixture of activity (which includes exercise and recreation), as well as rest and structured relaxation.'

If we are to lead healthier, more fulfilling lives, it is vital that we bring calm and tranquillity into our stress-filled times. Slowing down means that we function more effectively. Frantic, high-flying types – the ones who are only happy when they are doing five things at once and who denigrate relaxation as something kooky – should realise that being hyperactive is now considered deeply unfashionable. Serenity is a beauty imperative. But if switching off and relaxing seem an impossible task, even if you can only snatch a few moments in which to relax, you'll find that it gives you control over your life and looks.

Stress triggers what is known as a 'fight or flight' response, increasing the production of hormones, adrenalin, cortisol and non-adrenalin, which are responsible for sending your heart rate and blood pressure soaring. The body is equipped to deal with a certain amount of stress; however, continual stress, as a result of work overload, financial problems or other pressures, takes its toll on the body. Cells become filled with impurities, thus depriving the body of nutrients and resulting in spots, blotchy skin, eczema, dull hair and weak nails. Stress is also ageing: the cell-rebuilding process slows down, the body's water balance is disturbed and the rate of free-radical production increases. From a health aspect, stress inhibits breathing, breaks down the immune system and, as it creates more acid in the saliva, can even cause tooth decay.

But according to Dr Russell not all stress is bad: 'Too little stress leads to apathy and lack of motivation, so it's a case of keeping the stress levels balanced.' Nonetheless, he warns those whose stress levels are tilting towards the unhealthy to watch out for the danger signs, which include skin problems, tense muscles, moodiness, panic attacks, loss of libido, headaches, indigestion, lethargy, lack of concentration and insomnia. Dr Russell explains that even *he* cannot wave a magic wand: 'Realise your own limitations and change your lifestyle accordingly.'

If your usual way of dealing with stress is by smoking, knocking back a bottle of wine or indulging in some frantic retail therapy, firstly, turn to page 170 for stress-busting tips before endeavouring to bring some form of relaxation into your life. Plan a relaxation session at least twice a week: this could include taking up yoga, Pilates, t'ai chi, meditation or The Alexander Technique, which all help to relax the body, calm the mind and retrain you to breathe correctly. If all else fails, you could try a stress-management course: by dissecting and examining your own personal stress cycle you should come up with solutions. However, if you can practice Dr Russell's self-relaxation technique once a day, or even once a week, you might just find that stress becomes a thing of the past.

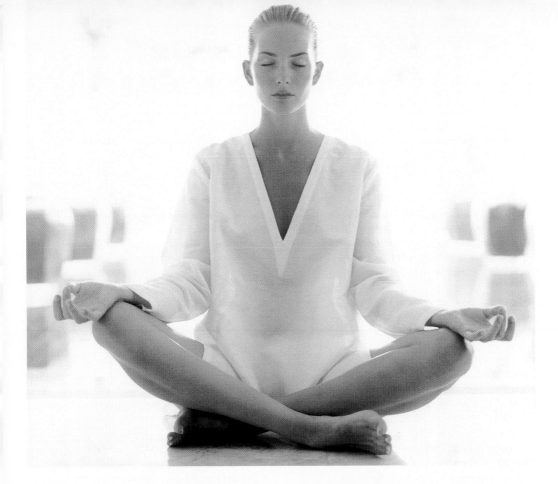

A SELF-RELAXATION TECHNIQUE

Dr Russell has devised a simple relaxation technique so easy that you can do it on the bus or train. When at home, find a quiet spot and play relaxing music if it helps. Enjoy your relaxed state for a minimum of five minutes, although in order to reap real benefits, twenty minutes is ideal. Practise it once a week and you'll soon start to feel more human again; practise it daily and you will feel like a new person. Start by lying down or sitting comfortably, with your back held straight.

• Close your eyes, take a deep breath and hold it for as long as possible. Exhale with a long, deep sigh and really try to feel that you are ridding yourself of stale air. Repeat.

• The second stage is to start breathing in a more relaxed way, from your diaphragm rather than taking shallow, rapid breaths from your chest. Inhale a long breath through your nose for approximately three to five seconds. Exhale by releasing your diaphragm slowly, for five to eight seconds, rather than forcing the air out.

• Breathe normally, allowing your mind and body to wind down into a comfortable state.

• Keeping your eyes closed, mentally scan your body for tension (perhaps your neck is stiff or your shoulders are tense). Now, each time you take a breath, as you exhale, use this breath to relax the parts of your body that need it.

• Finally, rejuvenate your mind by visualising the promise of a new future when you inhale, while when you exhale, imagine that you are ridding your body of all the stress and debris of life.

STRESS-BUSTERS

- **Spend a few moments each day in total piece and quiet:** do not talk, read, watch television, listen to the radio or do anything else to disrupt your tranquillity.

- **Avoid drinking coffee when under stress:** caffeine can increase your anxiety levels and make you nervy and jumpy. Sip calming herbal or fruit teas, such as camomile, lemonbalm or verbena, instead.

- **Read a novel:** this form of escapism will transport your mind into a different world and allow you less time for worrying.

Fiddle with a squeezy stress ball rather than biting your nails, picking your spots or lighting up yet another cigarette.

- **Don't rush:** get up fifteen minutes earlier each morning and always set aside extra time when travelling to an important appointment.

- **Clear your clutter:** a tidy desk is a tidy mind, so rid your desk, car and home of any unnecessary clutter. According to the principles of Feng Shui, this clears your energy fields and helps to release energy.

- **Don't take life so seriously:** if you strive for perfection, be it in your work, home or in the relationship with your partner, you will not only become frustrated and stressed, but it's unlikely that you will ever be satisfied. Remember that nobody is perfect.

- **Use a thermo-stress monitor:** if you register as stressed or tense on the monitor, follow a relaxation technique such as on page 169.

- **Calm, uplift and energise with colour therapy:** while red has an energising effect, orange uplifts you. The cool, calming colours are blues, purples and greens, which help lower blood pressure and reduce the heart rate, so surround yourself with these hues.

- **Play music:** you might prefer to listen to either gentle, relaxing music to soothe away the strains of the day, or else to something with a strong beat to lift your spirits.

- **Sing or hum:** by causing vibrations in your throat, singing or humming can relieve tension.

- **Pamper yourself:** have a relaxing treatment, such as a facial or massage, or simply lie back and relax in an aromatherapy bath for twenty minutes. Be sure to take the phone off the hook and lock the door.

- **Release neck tension:** by either doing a few simple neck exercises, giving yourself a massage, or by using finger pressure or a TENS machine (Transaltaneous Electrical Nerve Stimulation) on acupressure points, you can be your own therapist and ease away any tension.

- **Do something mindless:** constant mental stimulation can be stressful, so every once in a while take a break by doing nothing in particular or just vegetating in front of the TV.

- **Turn to nature:** take natural remedies to help to curb stress, anxiety or depression. St John's Wort, Rhodiola and sweet chestnut act as natural anti-depressants; Bach's Rescue Remedy is an instant pick-me-up; and Kava and valerian root are natural sedatives.

- **Slow down:** life shouldn't be just one big rush.

- **Massage away your stress:** a body massage encourages the muscles to relax, helps to disperse any knots, and soothes and calms the mind (see self-massage on page 173).

- **Unwind through relaxation:** autogenics is a form of relaxation, which works on the principle that you can instruct your body to experience such sensations as heaviness before progressively relaxing each part of the body. Another popular method of relaxation involves tensing and then releasing each part of your body in turn. Yoga, The Alexander Technique, Pilates, t'ai chi and mediation are also good methods of relaxation. Try de-stressing yourself with the aid of a self-relaxation breathing technique, such as the one on page 169.

- **Don't eat on the run:** this affects the digestion, which is disrupted during times of stress.

- **Sleep well:** stress disrupts the quality of sleep, which means that your body cannot rejuvenate itself properly (see page 167 for tips on how to get a good night's sleep).

- **Put your problems into perspective:** think about whether your problem is as bad as you are making it out to be – for example, will it really be the end of the world if you don't meet that deadline?

- **Step up your vitamin and mineral intake:** when you are under stress your body becomes depleted of nutrients, so make sure that you are eating healthily and take a good multi-vitamin-and-mineral supplement. Specific vitamins and minerals that are said to combat stress include vitamin C, vitamin B complex, vitamin B5, Siberian ginseng, calcium and magnesium (a natural tranquilliser).

- **Become organised:** write a 'to-do' list every day and cross out each task once you have completed it. Deal with administrative matters, like paying bills, as and when they arise, rather than letting them pile up on your table and in your mind.

- **Seek help:** to help manage stress, you could try various self-help therapies, such as Q-netics (a stress-release programme), stress-management courses and autogenic training.

- **Become active:** exercise has been shown to reduce stress, depression and anxiety. Thirty minutes of exercise three times a week will help to keep stress at bay. Go for a walk: the fresh air, combined with the exercise, will relax you.

- **Breathe deeply:** when you feel yourself getting stressed, breathe deeply and slowly from your diaphragm (see page 169).

- **Take up a pastime:** you might find that gardening, pottery or some other activity that you enjoy is incredibly therapeutic.

> **Laugh:** laughing is a natural tranquilliser – it stimulates the production of the feel-good hormones, endorphins, as well as of immunoglobin A, which strengthens the immune system.

- **De-stress yourself on the spot:** dab or spray on Origins' Peace of Mind, Crabtree & Evelyn's Relaxation Water Mist or a relaxing scent, such as Shiseido's Relaxing Fragrance, onto your wrist's pulse points. Put a drop or two of such calming essential oils as neroli, camomile, ylang-ylang, sandalwood, marjoram or lavender onto a tissue or cotton-wool ball and place it next to your bed or on your desk.

- **Keep work out of the bedroom:** your boudoir should be reserved for sleeping and making love, so don't attempt to read that report in bed!

- **Break routine:** a change is often as good as a rest, so plan a day's outing or weekend away. The fact that you are getting away from a stressful situation should alter your outlook.

- **Make love:** this instant tonic is one of the best tension busters.

MASSAGE

Imagine every inch of your body deliciously
relaxed – sound good? Then why not indulge in one of life's blissful experiences?

Once associated with back-street parlours and sleaze, these days massage is more likely to evoke images of health and well-being than sex. Back massages are now being given in offices, hospitals and coffee bars, as well as on aeroplanes. But this doesn't mean that the massage experience has evolved into a clinical procedure: stripping semi-naked and then being anointed with sweet-smelling oils is in itself decidedly sensual – this is way before the massage part has even started. Even a Chavutti-thirumal massage – in which the therapist kneads you with his or her feet – is guaranteed to send ripples of sensations through your body.

Massage is one of the best antidotes to stress and tension, but its benefits go further than this: an hour of escapism from the real world alters both your physical and mental state, and you should emerge feeling spiritually uplifted, totally relaxed and loose-limbed, having had the tension eased out of every inch of your muscles. But as Colin Crane, head masseur at Champneys Health Resort, points out, although the light, stroking type of massage administered by beauty therapists is relaxing, in order for you really to benefit from a treatment the masseur needs to apply a certain amount of pressure to work deep into the muscle. 'You need to rev up the circulation, expel toxins, oxygenate the cells and get the whole body moving,' says Colin, whose advice is to find a trained masseur or therapist who does more than just tickle you.

Since ancient times massage has been proved to be a great healer. But another advantage of having a professional massage is one that is often overlooked: being touched. The skin is not only a tactile organ, but we all crave the feeling of human connection created by a caressing touch, although this is something that is often missing in our lives. Besides, there's nothing quite like feeling the touch of experienced, oiled hands rubbing up and down your tense spine, pummelling deep into your knotted muscles, pressing the tender points on your face and gently stimulating your scalp.

There are now many different types of massage on offer, from the simple, back-and-neck method to aromatherapy, holistic, shiatsu, chua-ka deep-tissue, Thai, Swedish, Tibetan, Indonesian, Indian (head), Chavutti-thirumal and tui-na, to name but a few. The benefits differ from massage to massage: while a Swedish massage, for example, leaves you feeling invigorated and bursting with energy, an aromatherapy treatment can be so relaxing that it sends you to sleep.

The person who administers the massage is another important factor to consider (I personally prefer the strong pummelling of a male masseur to the softer, more soothing touch of a masseuse). Try out a few different massage techniques and you'll be sure to stumble across one that really works for you. If possible, have a massage at least once a month.

SELF BODY MASSAGE

With the help of Colin Crane, Champneys Health Resort's head of massage, here is a self-massage that will benefit your whole body by improving your circulation and releasing the tension in your muscles. Rather than just stroking the skin, this massage involves administering slow, deep, gliding movements using a certain amount of pressure. Combine these movements with pummelling and kneading actions using your fingers, thumbs and knuckles, as well as performing a press-release action with your fingers. If an area feels sore, use the press-release method until the pain eases.

If you only have olive oil in the house, this is fine; you can always add a couple of drops of your favourite essential oil to it. Alternatively, if you want to invest in a good massage oil, try Philosophy's Physical Therapy or E'spa's Restorative Massage Oil. Start by relaxing for a few moments while lying on your back, either on a bed, mat or towel placed on the floor. Make sure that the room is warm and, with the exception of the area that you are treating, keep your body covered up with a towel.

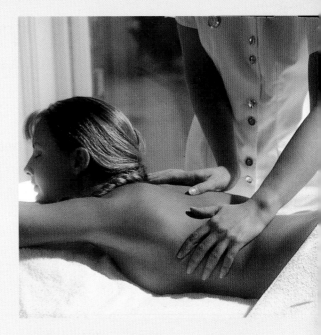

- **Feet:** sit up and bend your legs so that you can comfortably reach your feet. With your thumbs, using a press-release action, massage the sole and top of each foot and knead between your toes. Squeeze your toes between your fingers and thumb. When you reach your ankles, use small finger rotations.
- **Calves:** keeping your knees bent, using gliding, upward movements, smooth oil along your calves and up the front of your legs.
- **Knees:** in order to be able to gain access to your knee, keep your leg bent and turn your foot outwards before kneading each side of the knee with your thumbs. Now turn your foot inwards and repeat the massage.
- **Thighs:** sweep your hands up the front of each thigh in large, gliding movements (it is advisable to use gentle pummelling movements on the back of your thighs because of the hamstring).
- **Buttocks:** kneel or stand. Start by kneading around the top of the hamstring (just under each buttock) and then pummel the buttock itself.

- **Back:** massaging the whole of your back is a bit tricky, but you can work on your lower back and shoulders quite effectively. Sit or kneel, whichever is most comfortable. Start by kneading your lower back around the muscles located on either side of the vertebrae (use both hands simultaneously). For your shoulders, reach one hand to the opposite shoulder and glide it across, using circular rotations. Repeat on each shoulder.
- **Neck:** using the press-release action, rotate your fingers around each side of your neck.
- **Abdomen:** lie down on your back and sweep your hands across your stomach in gliding, circular movements.
- **Chest:** knead between your breasts with your knuckles. Smooth oil onto your breasts and circle them, using gliding movements.
- **Arms:** lie down on your back, or sit if you prefer. Knead your lower arms, working towards your elbows. When you reach your upper arms, use gliding movements.
- **Hands and wrists:** use circular actions around the wrist joint, changing to the press-release method on your palms. Move on to the fingers and, using your thumb and forefinger, stroke down each finger towards the nail.

HEALTH SPAS

There is a place that comes close to paradise – a tranquil haven
a million miles from reality, where you arrive feeling frazzled and depart having refreshed
and rejuvenated your mind, body and soul.

Having been pampered, pummelled and perfumed at various spas, I must declare that escaping to a spa, health farm, retreat, hydro – or whatever other fancy name the resort may call itself – is one of life's luxuries. And if we are to disperse some of that pent-up tension from which we are suffering, living as we do in this fast-track world, a spa break looks increasingly like becoming a necessity rather than an indulgence. Even a day's visit will leave you feeling relaxed, revitalised and ready to face life's challenges. But the benefits go further still: while unwinding in one of these heavenly oases, you can't help but start to rethink your lifestyle. And if your visit inspires you to take just one step towards looking and feeling better, be it by eating less sugar or giving up smoking, it will have been worth every penny.

Forget the conventional, austere health-farm image, in which white-coated types doused you in ice-cold water and denied you any real food.

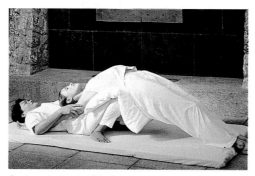

One-to-one treatment at Chiva-Som.

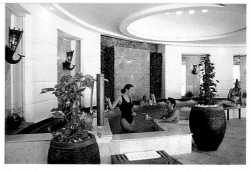

A dip in the spa at the exotic Chiva-Som Health Resort in Thailand.

Over the past few years spas have undergone a total revamp, shifting their emphasis from administering boarding-school-style punishment to pampering and de-stressing their clients and, at a few select resorts, offering spiritual enlightenment, too. Luxury body-wraps have replaced Spartan, slimming treatments, while calorie-counting regimes have been swapped for Michelin-star-rated cuisine. Some spas, like Clinique La Prairie in Switzerland, take their beauty treatments a step further by offering a range of anti-ageing procedures.

You can even holiday in the ultimate dream location while enjoying the benefits of a spa. Most resorts offer every activity under the sun, including golf, tennis, archery, squash, mountain biking and, at the beach resorts, such water sports as windsurfing, catamaran sailing and scuba diving – ideal for entertaining your other half while you lie cocooned in a blissful, marine-algae wrap.

SPA DIRECTORY

Spas differ. Aside from such purpose-built health resorts like Champneys, there are many five-star hotels world-wide, such as Turnbury, Le Sport, The Paris Ritz and Chewton Glen, which have fabulous spas on site. There are also one-stop urban spas for city-dwellers, as well as mini-spas, which offer more than a health club or beauty salon. Here is the international pick of the bunch. Before each of the numbers first dial the international dialing code and the country code.

England
Aveda Urban Retreat, London
Tel: 0171 201 8610

Cedar Falls Health Farm
Tel: 01823 433233

Champneys Health Resort
Tel: 01442 291111

Chewton Glen Hotel and
Country Club
Tel: 01425 275341

The Dorchester Spa, London
Tel: 0171 495 7335

Greyshot Hall Health &
Fitness Retreat
Tel: 01428 604331

Ragdale Hall Health Hydro
Tel: 01664 434831

Shambhala Centre for
Spiritual Growth and Healing
Tel: 01458 831797

Scotland
Turnbury Hotel and Spa
Tel: 01655 331000

Australia
The Hyatt Regency Coolum
Beach Spa, Queensland
Tel: 75 4461234

Austria
Grand Hotel Sauerhof, Vienna
Tel: 2252 412510

France
Hélianthal Spa, St Jean de Luis
Tel: 559 515151

Ritz Hotel Health Club, Paris
Tel: 143 163060

Monaco
Thermes Marines Spa, Monaco
Tel: 92 164040

Germany
Brenner's Park Hotel and Spa,
Baden-Baden
Tel: 72 2190 00

Italy
Grotta Giusti Spa, Tuscany
Tel: 0572 51008

St Lucia
Le Sport Hotel and Spa
Tel: 450 8551

Sweden
Selma Lagerlof Hotel and Spa,
Sunne
Tel: 565 16608

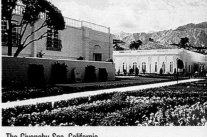

The Givenchy Spa, California

Switzerland
Clinique La Prairie, Montreux
Tel: 21989 3311

Thailand
Chiva-Som Health Resort
Tel: 32 536536

United Arab Emirates
Cleopatra's Spa, Dubai
Tel: 43244757

USA
The Aveda Institute,
Minneapolis
Tel: 612 378 7400

Bliss Spa, New York
Tel: 212 219 8970

Chopra Center for Well
Being, California
Tel: 619 551 7788

Givenchy Hotel and Spa,
California
Tel: 760 770 5000

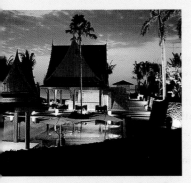

Sunrise over Chiva-Som and the Gulf of Siam.

A DIARY OF MY SPA EXPERIENCE

DAY ONE

In need of some intense pampering, I head off to sample the spa experience for myself. I arrive at Greyshot Hall, a beautiful, old stately home, with ivy crawling up its red-brick walls and serene, country-house-style décor. I can best describe this place as luxury hotel meets beauty clinic, with a health-cum-country-club feel to it. There is an unmistakable feeling of tranquillity about the place, and when I spot the guests wafting around in fluffy white bathrobes and slippers, I realise how far removed we are from reality.

Swim in the pool: there's no time to waste, so as I wait for my companion to arrive I swim a few lengths of the pool, basking in the fact that I have three days of shameless self-indulgence ahead of me. Full of apologies for being late, Julie arrives looking frazzled and sounding stressed, but as soon as she exchanges her business suit for a freshly-laundered bathrobe, she looks like a new woman.

Lunch: no boring old lettuce leaves here, although a peek into the light-diet room tells us that for the calorie-counters the food is rather less inspiring. With not an ounce of guilt, we heap spoonfuls of delicious, yet healthy, hot and cold food from the buffet onto our plates. As our dessertspoons clink into our empty bowls, we both feel satisfied, knowing that every mouthful has been highly nutritious and not in the least bit fattening.

Health check: the obligatory health check is carried out by a caring nurse with a soothing voice, who weighs me, asks me lots of questions about my health, and then suggests the treatments that she thinks I would benefit from most during my stay.

Splash class in the pool: this involves ring-a-roses-style movements and a weird exercise in which we have to jump around with a float between our legs. Lots of fun, but not exactly what I'd call exercise.

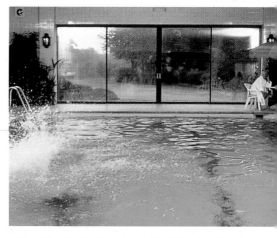

Within minutes of arriving I have stripped off and plunged into the pool.

Fitness assessment in the gym: after a chat with trainer Ravi, I am under no illusion that I will become superfit in three days. Nonetheless, this is the spur I need, so Ravi shows me both a fitness regime that I can continue with at home and a workout using the gym equipment.

Oriental wisdom: in a dimly-lit room suffused with spiritual music, I experience a wonderful combination of shiatsu, tui-na Chinese massage, reflexology and aromatherapy, which makes for the perfect massage – relaxing, stimulating and healing at the same time. When I return to our room, Julie is reclined on her bed recovering from her holistic-massage experience. 'Had the masseuse been male it would have been *too* much,' she says wistfully. I must try this one next time!

Dinner: candlelight, waiter service and a gourmet menu – everything you'd expect from a first-class restaurant, with only one difference: the dress code is nothing but a bathrobe!

Midnight rendezvous: to the insomniacs' room, where tea, coffee and every imaginable herbal infusion is available day and night. You can even have a biscuit or two if you ask nicely.

DAY TWO

Heat treatment: at 8am, still sleepy and bleary-eyed, I am placed in a steam cabinet and then left to bake for ten minutes. Too much of a wimp to jump into the ice-cold plunge pool, I opt for a luke warm shower. As I step out, I am wrapped in a warm towel, handed a glass of refreshing lime juice and then ushered into the relaxation room, where I am tucked up in a bed and left until my masseur is ready for me.

Massage: I plump for a male masseur and, when a fellow female guest comes out of the massage room with a big smile on her face, I praise myself for having made the right choice. However, once the pummelling starts – and boy does he pummel – I long for the soft, caressing touch of a masseuse. But after a few 'ouches' and groans, I relax into a deep slumber knowing that if this doesn't shift my cellulite – nothing will.

Breakfast: who said anything about starving? Then again, mushrooms on brown toast is the closest you'll get to a full English fry-up. Never mind – there is a delicious aray of exotic fruits, yoghurt and muesli, together with plenty of hot tea, toast and home-made marmalade.

Golf tuition: novice that I am, I am most impressed that after forty-five minutes on the driving range I can actually hit the ball.

Lunch: I'm already munching a crispbread when Julie arrives, red-faced and accompanied by a male admirer whom she met during circuit-training in the gym. This reafirms my point that spas are not only crawling with women.

Meet with the dietician: Paula designs a healthy-eating plan to boost my immune system. Good news: I'm still allowed a cake each afternoon!

Reiki: this can best be described as the laying-on of hands. Admittedly, I find it relaxing, but that pretty much sums it up. It certainly isn't the 'spiritual' experience that Julie had a few hours earlier. (I'm beginning to think Julie is having all the fun around here!) Mind you, it just goes to show that what one person considers bliss, another finds boring.

Evening fun: the entertainment on offer is 'fun and games' in the lounge. However, the movie channel takes priority.

DAY THREE

Early morning walk: while Julie struts off for the one-hour power-walk, I join the 'gentle' meander, which I soon realise is for geriatrics.

Cranial osteopathy: having woken up with a head-splitting migraine, this is the treatment I'm looking forward to the most.

Thalgo collagen facial: a luxurious, hour-and-a-half-long treatment that promises to make me look five years younger. When at lunch, Julie's admirer tells me that I look fifteen years old, I know it has worked.

Lunch: We decide to sit at the large table (common at most spas) reserved for those who have come alone and want to meet others. I chat to fellow guests to find out their motives for coming here, which appear to be a mixture of – get fit, lose weight and de-stress. I soon suss out the naughty ones who have smuggled in chocolate – the ultimate spa sin!

Algae body wrap: as I lie defenceless and naked on a bench, the therapist sloughs off my dead skin with a salt scrub and then embalms me in a seaweedy gunge. This stuff smells so strongly of fish that had there been any spa cats they would have been drooling in this room. I am then wrapped in a thermal blanket and left to boil in the bag for ten minutes. I nod off.

Time to leave: as we drive away, we feel the most relaxed that we have felt in years.

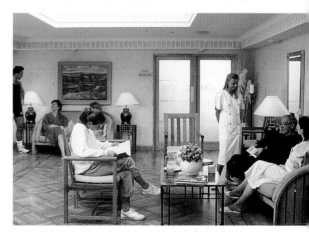

Waiting in the spa atrium to be called for my massage.

EATING FOR BEAUTY

If you want a clearer, brighter complexion, glossy hair, strong nails, no cellulite and a slim physique, you need to eat a healthy, balanced diet which includes a variety of nutritious foods to enable your body to absorb the vital nutrients that it requires.

The nutritional buzz words are moderation and balance. Lyndel Costain, a consultant dietician and health columnist, believes that although you should eat healthily, no food should be strictly forbidden. Paula Gilbert, head of nutrition at Greyshot Hall Health and Fitness Retreat, looks upon the naughty treats as compensation: 'If you've eaten well all week, you can treat yourself to a piece of chocolate or something else you fancy,' she says. My personal treat of the week is an Irish coffee; it contains all the 'bad' boys: caffeine, sugar, alcohol and cream. But it's delicious and, as it's the weekend, I'm allowed to bend the rules. Eat sensibly, not rigidly, and allow yourself the occasional indulgence, because being overvirtuous is boring, and boring is not beautiful!

HEALTHY-EATING CHECKLIST

- **Eat regularly:** consume three meals a day. Don't skip breakfast – it's vital if you want to kick-start your metabolism and avoid mid-morning cravings. Eat every three to five hours.
- **Eat freshly prepared wholefoods:** the food that you eat should be as close to its natural state as possible. Processed foods have little nutritional value and are laced with saturated fats, chemical additives, preservatives, sugar and salt.
- **Choose unrefined in preference to refined food:** eat rice, pasta and bread in their brown, unrefined state instead of white alternatives.
- **Eat organic:** unlike non-organic produce, these foods are not contaminated with chemicals, fertilisers, hormones and pesticides.

- **Ignore the food myths and fad diets:** 'Eating starts becoming complicated and confusing when you worry about things like eating fruit at certain times or eating protein separately from carbohydrates,' says Lyndel.
- **Cook lightly:** stir-fry, bake, grill, steam or poach food as opposed to barbecuing, boiling, chargrilling or deep-frying it.
- **Eat five portions of fresh fruit and vegetables a day:** fruit and vegetables are laden with nutrients and antioxidants and are also cleansing and energy-giving. Try to eat a variety of fruit and vegetables, and eat them raw wherever possible.
- **Include essential fatty acids (EFAs) in your diet:** found in oils and fats, EFAs are vital to a healthy body as they help to build cell membranes and condition skin, hair and nails from within. The beneficial EFAs are contained in the polyunsaturated and monounsaturated fats that are prevalent in vegetable oils (including walnut, linseed, grape-seed, olive, sesame and avocado), oily fish, vegetables, seeds, nuts and whole grains. The key sources include linolenic acid (found in green, leafy vegetables); linoleic acid (which is most abundant in sesame, grape-seed and sunflower oil); and omega 3s (prevalent in oily fish). To ensure that you eat adequate amounts of EFAs, use EFA-rich oils in their unrefined forms as salad dressings daily, and eat oily fish twice a week.
- **Supplement your food:** there are arguments for and against vitamin and mineral supplements. Supplement sceptics believe that we should be getting adequate nutrients from our food, while those who are in favour of supplements stress that we need to compensate for our poor eating habits: eating convenience food and eating on the run. If you are taking individual vitamin or mineral supplements, always combine them with a good multi-vitamin-and-mineral. Paula suggests buying the best you can afford.

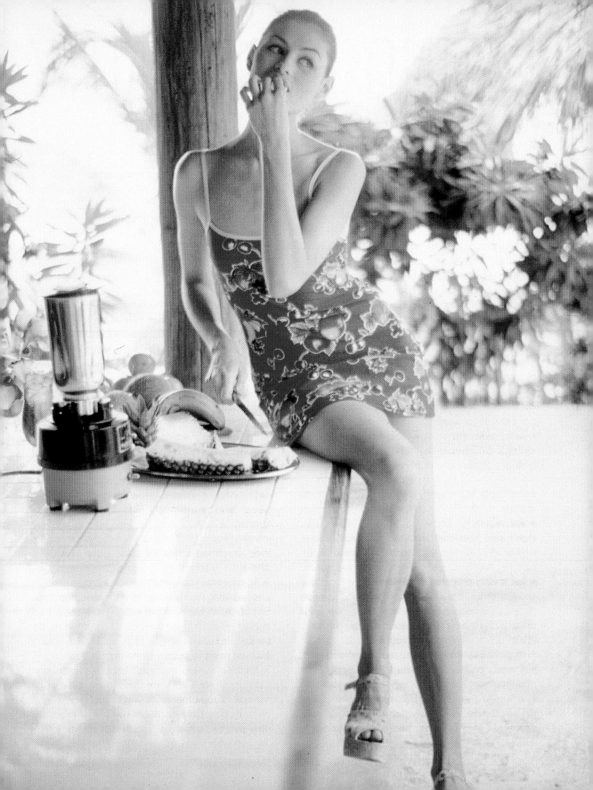

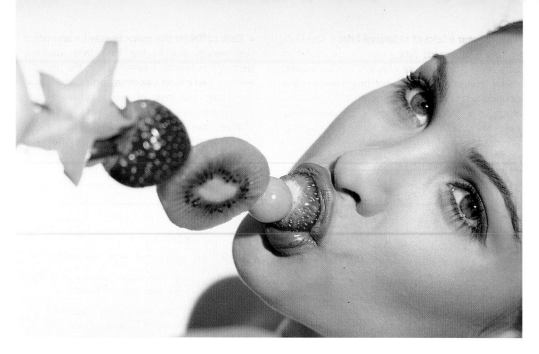

- **Divide your plate:** at Champneys Health Resort the plates are marked with dividing lines to ensure that guests are eating a balanced meal. You can improvise at home by dividing your plate into three sections: twenty-five per cent for protein – such as fish, meat, beans and cheese; twenty-five per cent for carbohydrates – like rice, bread or pasta (brown wherever possible); and fifty per cent for veg or salad.
- **Introduce beans and pulses to your diet:** these are an excellent source of fibre, amino acids, vitamins and minerals.
- **Increase your fibre intake:** abundant in fruit, vegetables, beans, pulses and whole grains, fibre is mainly found in the peel of fruit and vegetables and in the outer layers of grains. It's essential to eat plenty of fibre-rich food in order to aid healthy digestion, prevent constipation and eliminate waste matter. In beauty terms, a sluggish digestion can result in dull, greyish skin, spots, under-eye shadows and puffiness.
- **Don't overlook nuts and seeds:** small, but highly nutritious, seeds like pumpkin, sesame and sunflower can be sprinkled onto salads, cereals and sandwich fillings, whereas nuts can be eaten as a healthy snack.

THE 'BAD' BOYS

- **Eliminate sugar:** the chocoholics and sweet-toothed among you will be disappointed to know that sugar is not only of no nutritional value but, what's worse, is actually bad for you. The obviously negative effects of sugar are tooth decay and weight gain but, as too much sugar can block the colon, making it impermeable to nutrients, it can have a knock-on effect on the skin, hair and nails. Avoid fizzy drinks, sweet snacks, cakes, biscuits, jam, condiments and sugar-coated cereals, and do not use sugar to sweeten your tea or coffee. Healthier alternatives include honey, fructose (the sugar found in fruit) and molasses.
- **Omit salt:** beware of oversprinkling salt on your food because it can affect your looks. Salt prevents the kidneys from filtering fluid correctly and can therefore cause water retention, leading to puffy eyes and even cellulite.
- **Moderate your alcohol intake:** The dehydration that is responsible for your hangover, also causes premature ageing by depleting the skin of moisture. Excessive amounts of alcohol will deplete the body of vital nutrients.

• **Lower your intake of saturated fats:** a diet high in 'bad' (saturated) fats – which are found in fatty meat and dairy products, such as butter, full-fat milk and cream – not only piles on the pounds and causes spots and cellulite, but also clogs up our bodies. Lyndel advises lowering our saturated-fat intake. But rather than cutting fat out of our diets (we all need a certain amount of fat), she suggests drinking semi-skimmed rather than skimmed milk and opting for low-fat as opposed to fat-free foods.

• **Curb caffeine:** this quick fix may be an instant pick-me-up, but in the long term caffeine destroys nutrients, overstimulates the nervous system, can cause insomnia and irritability, and increases the risk of more severe health problems, such as high blood pressure. Coffee, tea, chocolate and cola drinks all contain caffeine, but coffee has the highest level of it; (decaffeinated is not necessarily healthier as it contains other toxic ingredients that are also stimulants, such as benzoic acid).

THE KEY BEAUTY NUTRIENTS

Nutrients	What they do	Sources
Vitamin A	Repairs skin tissue and improves texture	Eggs, liver, butter and cod liver oil
Betacarotene	An antioxidant which helps to scavenge free radicals	Yellow/orange fruits and vegetables, like apricots and carrots
Vitamin C	An antioxidant, it also aids collagen synthesis and has healing properties	Citrus fruits, kiwis, cranberries, broccoli, brussel sprouts, blackcurrants and watercress
Vitamin E	An antioxidant, it also repairs cell membranes and improves the skin's elasticity	Avocados, wheatgerm, nuts, seeds, eggs, sunflower and cornflower oils
Vitamin B complex	This assists the skin's tissue function, boosts circulation and balances oil production	Cereals, brewer's yeast, liver, egg yolks, whole grains and sardines
Amino acids	Maintain healthy skin and have skin-repairing properties	Meat, oats, beans, wheatgerm, lentils, tofu, eggs, milk and cheese
Essential fatty acids	Lubricate the skin, hair and nails from within	Green, leafy vegetables, vegetable oils and oily fish
Enzymes	These strengthen collagen and elastin fibres	Pineapples and papayas
Selenium	An antioxidant which helps mop up free radicals and maintains skin tissue	Brewer's yeast, avocados, whole grains, fish, nuts, seafood and bread
Iron	This oxygenates cells	Liver, red meat, green, leafy vegetables (especially spinach), fish and dried fruit
Sulphur	Helps create keratin, a protein substance necessary for healthy skin, nails and hair	Shellfish, eggs, peas, kidney beans, poultry, nuts and milk
Zinc	Prevents stretchmarks and white spots on nails, and improves skin elasticity	Seafood, wheatgerm, organ meat, cereals, mushrooms, milk and sunflower seeds
Magnesium	Known as nature's tranquilliser	Seafood, soya, beans, green, leafy vegetables, bran, oats, nuts and whole grains

SVELTE WITHOUT STARVING

Wouldn't you love to be able to eat large, appetising plates of
food without piling on the pounds? Here's how to stay svelte the healthy way.

Food is fuel, so deprivation ultimately means starvation. When you diet, not only are you starving your stomach of food, but you are also depriving every living cell in your body of nutrients; so forget about strict diets and obsessive calorie-counting. According to consultant dietician and health columnist Lyndel Costain, the best way to in which to stay slim or lose weight is to eat a healthy well-balanced diet rather than resorting to dieting: 'If you tell yourself you're on a diet, psychologically you will feel deprived and are more likely to crave bad foods and end up bingeing.'

SLIMMING STRATAGIES

by Lyndel Costain

Successful slimmers are usually those who develop their own strategies. Here are my strategies for success, together with key steps towards losing weight.
• Weight-loss strategies include: viewing weight-control as a long-term commitment and setting realistic goals; realising that there will be inevitable ups and downs; keeping a food diary to monitor your eating habits; building some extra activity into your schedule that you can keep up; avoiding using food for comfort and finding other ways with which to cope with stressful problems; eating more fruit and vegetables and lower-fat foods; and praising yourself for any successes.
• The basis for all these weight-loss strategies is that you, the individual, are in charge, so tailor them to suit yourself.
• Think long term and be realistic about how much weight to lose and how quickly. Use your food diary before making any lifestyle changes and then take them one at a time.

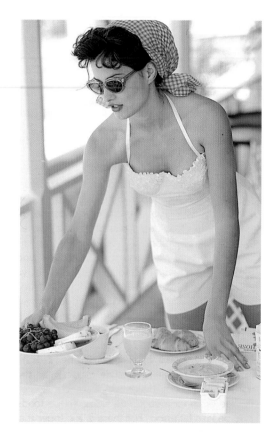

• If your weight starts creeping up, don't panic: use the strategies listed in my first point to help you get back on track.
• Don't think that you have to do it alone: success is more likely if you have support that suits you, for example, from a health professional, a responsible slimming group or publication, or a good friend or partner (people who are severely obese are always advised to seek medical advice).

A DOZEN TACTICS TO HELP YOU TO STAY SLIM WITHOUT DIETING

1 **Savour and enjoy:** when eating, slow down and savour every bite. Wolfing down mouthfuls of food is unlikely to leave you feeling satisfied and could bring about digestive problems. By chewing your food slowly, you will enjoy its flavour and are likely to feel satisfied with less.

2 **Stick to a plan:** plan what and when you are going to eat (this includes snacks). This way you are less likely to raid the biscuit tin when you have a food craving.

3 **Fill your plate with appetising food:** pile up your plate with healthy food, especially salads and vegetables, which you can eat in abundance. By taking longer to plough through your meal you will feel full and, in psychological terms, will think that you've eaten a large meal. Another mind trick is to fool yourself into thinking that you've eaten more by using a smaller plate. When preparing food, make it look as appetising as possible: a plate of uninspiring lettuce leaves is enough to make anyone dive for a gooey cake.

4 **Don't be fooled by diet foods:** be it 'light' mayonnaise or 'diet' chocolate mousse, all the rich, naughty foods that we love come in lighter, fat-free or sugar-reduced versions. These foods may be less fattening, but there is a danger that you will pile twice as much onto your plate.

5 **Don't go for more than five hours without eating:** if you go for too long without food your blood-sugar level drops, leaving you feeling lethargic, so you could end up eating far more than you would have done in the first place. 'This can spell disaster,' says Greyshot Hall Health and Fitness Retreat's nutritionist, Paula Gilbert. 'If you haven't eaten enough earlier in the day, you are more likely to binge.'

6 **Drink a glass of water thirty minutes before a meal:** this will fill you up, which means that you are more likely to eat less.

7 **Say 'no' to fancy extras:** garlic bread, crisps, canapés and rolls with butter are tempting, but such extras can often be more fattening than the meal itself. If you need to nibble, replace crisps with pre-dinner snacks like unsalted nuts or raw vegetables dipped in humus.

8 **Visualise a slimmer you:** each time you find yourself reaching for a bar of chocolate, stop. Instead, visualise a slimming goal, such as looking sylph-like in your favourite outfit.

9 **Snack healthily:** if you're used to indulging yourself with high-fat snacks and can't fight your food cravings, snack on fruit, vegetables, dried fruit, nuts, raisins or low-fat yoghurt. To avoid temptation, don't keep any sweets, biscuits, chocolates or other naughty snacks at home.

10 **Become active:** combine a healthy diet with regular exercise to keep yourself trim and control any food cravings. If you haven't got the time or money to join a health club, exercise at home.

11 **Treat yourself:** set yourself goals and then, when you've achieved them, award yourself with a treat. If you're a compulsive chocolate lover, and have managed to go without any for a week, reward yourself with your favourite chocolate bar.

12 **Satisfy your sweet tooth:** eliminating sugar from your diet doesn't mean that you have to deprive yourself of sweet-tasting foods. If you have an urge for sugary stuff, eat foods containing natural sugar, such as fruit and honey, as these are healthier than refined sugar.

SPA RECIPES

CHIVA-SOM: CARROT CINNAMON CAKE

A delicious, yet healthy, cake from this heavenly resort, which was developed by its masterchef Andrew Jacka.

340g flour
250g brown sugar
2 teaspoons baking powder
150ml apple juice
4 egg whites
240g carrots, grated
50g raisins

Preheat the oven to 160°C/310°F/gas mark 2. Mix the flour, brown sugar and baking powder together. Stir in the apple juice, egg whites, carrots and raisins. Pour into a ten-inch cake ring and bake for thirty to thirty-five minutes.

CLINIQUE LA PRAIRIE: PEARS WITH RED WINE AND THYME

Elfried Blaes, the head chef at this Swiss spa, has created a wonderful dessert with which to impress your dinner guests. (Serves 4.)

4 large ripe pears
300ml red wine
200ml orange juice
4 cooked twigs thyme
1 measure agar-agar or cornstarch
4 tablespoons sweetening powder

Peel the pears, leaving the stems on. Bring the red wine, orange juice and thyme to the boil in a saucepan. Add the pears to the boiling liquid, reduce the heat and cook on a low heat until they are tender. Remove the liquid from the heat and let it cool. Remove the pears from the juice, cut them in half or in slices and arrange them on serving plates which have a raised rim. Add the agar-agar or cornstarch to the liquid, bring it quickly to the boil and reduce to one third, add the sweetener and pour over the pears. Decorate with the cooked branches of thyme.

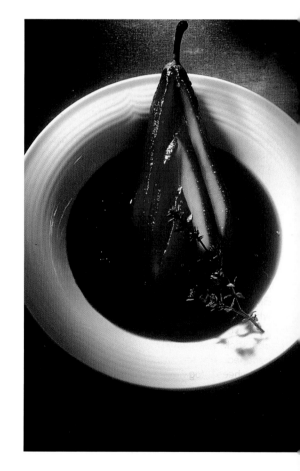

CHAMPNEYS: FETA CHEESE, LEEK, POTATO AND YOGHURT TARTLETS

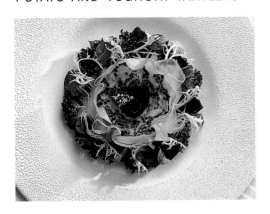

From this world-famous spa come these mouth-watering tartlets, created by chef Adam Palmer, which are ideal for lunch or a light supper. (Serves 4.)

4 sheets ready-made filo pastry
1 egg white
1 small leek, finely diced
1 clove garlic, finely diced
4 small new potatoes, lightly scrubbed and grated
55g feta cheese
150ml low-fat natural yoghurt
2 eggs
1 teaspoon walnut oil
1 bunch chives, finely chopped
A selection of salad leaves, torn
Sea salt and freshly milled black pepper
Marjoram flowers and pickled-walnut halves for garnish

Preheat the oven to 190°C/375°F/gas mark 5. Brush two sheets of filo pastry with a little egg white and line four three-inch tartlet moulds with two layers of pastry. Sweat the leek in a non-stick pan with the garlic until it has softened. Mix the potatoes, leeks, garlic and feta cheese together and place in the pastry cases. Mix the yoghurt with the eggs, add the chives and season to taste. Pour into the pastry cases and bake for fifteen minutes. Gently ease the cases from the moulds and serve with salad leaves tossed in walnut oil.

GIVENCHY HOTEL AND SPA: CHILLED GAZPACHO SOUP WITH A SERRANO FLAN

A delicious recipe from the resort's chef, Luis Garcia, which will make any lunch or dinner party a big success. (Serves 6.)
Ingredients for the gazpacho soup
½ green bell pepper, cored
½ red bell pepper, cored
3 tablespoons cucumber, peeled and chopped
3 tablespoons white onion, chopped
1 tablespoon celery, chopped
2 cups tomato juice
1 cup V8 juice
75g white-wine vinegar
Salt and freshly ground pepper
Garnish
1 tablespoon of green bell pepper, peeled, seeded and diced
1 tablespoon of red bell pepper, peeled, seeded and diced
½ cup bread crutons
Preparation for the gazpacho soup
Combine the peppers, cucumber, onion, celery with the V8 and tomato juice. Add the vinegar and season to taste with salt and pepper. Garnish with the bread croutons and bell peppers. Chill for at least eight hours.
Ingredients for the Serrano flan
1 pinch Serrano pepper, seeded and chopped
1 teaspoon chives, sliced
1 cup milk
1 whole egg
1 egg yolk
1 clove garlic, diced
Salt and freshly ground pepper
Preparation for the Serrano flan
Preheat the oven to 180°C/350°F/gas mark 4. Bring the milk to the boil. Combine the remaining ingredients in a bowl and pour into the boiling milk. Pour into an oven-proof form and place in a *bain-marie* or hot-water bath in the oven. Poach for thirty minutes. Allow the flan to cool and then dice it into small pieces.

SEX FOR BEAUTY

From aphrodisiacs and love potions to a
supersperm serum – here's how to become beautiful the sexual way.

• A sexual glow: Better than the most expensive cosmetic blush, the post-orgasmic flush leaves women looking rosy-cheeked and at their most beautiful. Next time that you make love, look at yourself in the mirror afterwards. Now try to create that look with make-up!

• Supersperm serum: Fresh semen rivals the best ingredients of cosmetic science as one of the most nourishing facial serums around. For a firmer, softer skin, spread it on your face and, just like a face mask, leave it on for ten minutes before washing it off with a foaming cleanser and plenty of warm water.

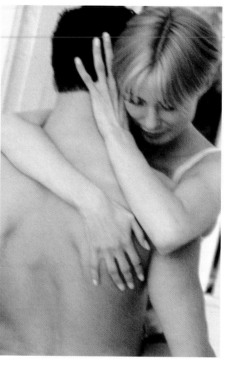

• Go solo: You don't have to be with a partner to benefit from sex. Admittedly, your physical workout may not be quite as thorough, but you can still reap the beauty rewards from both arousal and climax. Indulge in uninhibited fantasies and, if required, enlist the help of erotica. Judi Keshet-Orr, a psychosexual therapist, suggests treating masturbation as sex for one rather than a rushed stimulation session.

• Orgasmic relaxation: If you find it difficult to relax, let an orgasm do it for you. During arousal, your body produces the natural amphetamine PEA. You tend to breathe more deeply, which also aids relaxation. This is followed by an even deeper state of relaxation and finally a release of mental and physical tension directly after climax, which leaves you with that feeling of post-coital euphoria. So take advantage of this natural relaxant by letting your body become totally limp and enjoying this semi-hypnotic state. (Don't worry if you do not reach the point of orgasm: both the arousal stage and the 'plateau' phase – the feeling of being in limbo – before climax are just as beneficial.)

• A facial workout: If you yearn for chiselled cheekbones but don't have time for a full facial workout, there's nothing better than oral sex for toning and shaping your face.

• Silky-soft skin: When you make love, the physical activity stimulates the blood circulation, which brings a higher degree of oxygenation to your cells. Regular sex can therefore give you a softer, smoother and more youthful-looking complexion.

- **Tasty turn-ons:** Most of us would be positively turned off by powdered rhinoceros horn, Spanish fly and prairie oysters (bulls testicles), but aside from being from quite revolting and hard to find, Spanish fly, for example, contains dangerous chemicals. But take heart, there are plenty of more common aphrodisiacs to indulge in, such as chocolate, honey, aloe vera, celery, shiitake mushrooms, ginseng, avocado, nuts, dates, figs, papaya, royal jelly, ginger and passionfruit.

- **Sexy smiles:** Smiling is sexy and, according to dentist to the stars, Dr Marc Lowenberg, a sexy smile is defined by healthy-looking, white teeth, and also, a mouth in which the two front teeth are slightly longer than the adjacent ones. This can be achieved by cosmetic dentistry using veneers and reshaping but, as Dr Lowenberg points out: 'What looks sexy on one person could resemble rabbit teeth on another.'

- **Sensual tresses:** Your primary physical sexual attributes are your genitals, but as these cannot be flaunted, use one of your secondary sexual characteristics – your hair – to both attract and pull off a new sexy identity. A sexy mane is defined by silky, healthy-looking hair that swings with movement, so get your tresses in tiptop condition. To morph into a siren, wear your hair in a shoulder-skimming style, with a flirty fringe or, as stylist Colin Gold suggests: 'Have your hair styled in a slightly unstructured way so that it falls softly onto the face or over the eyes, for naturally sexy hair is "peep through" hair.' Finally, colour can transform the girl-next-door-type into a sex kitten.

- **Seductive eyes:** A key instrument in the art of seduction are the eyes. When you are attracted to someone your pupils dilate, making your eyes look larger and more attractive. In order to create seductive eyes artificially, elongate them by drawing a fine line along the upper lashes, taking it from the point above the centre of your pupil to the outer corner of your eyes. To emphasise your eyes further, give yourself luscious lashes by using an eyelash curler before strategically placing one or two individual false eyelashes at the upper outer corner of each eye.

- **Sexy clothes:** Flaunt your femininity by dressing sexily. High heels, skimpy dresses, push-up bras, mini-skirts, boots and sheer fabrics are the obvious sexy items, but remember that one way of sabotaging a potentially sexy look is to overdo it. So be subtle: a glimpse of cleavage or midriff, or an accidental flash of leg, is all that it takes. Underwear (such as little slips or bras) worn as outerwear can be deeply sexy, as long as it's not so transparent that it reveals all.

- **Body language:** A primal way of showing interest in someone is to stand close to them. Your stance is also a giveaway: thrusting your breasts or hips slightly forward spells interest. If you want to master the body language of a temptress, the trick is all in your posture: good carriage imparts confidence, which is in itself decidedly alluring.

- **Aphrodisiac aromatherapy:** Improve your sexual appetite with the help of the intoxicating vapours of such essential oils as ylang-ylang, rose, geranium, benzoin, clary sage and sandalwood. Place the oils in a burner, add a few drops to an unfragranced body lotion or give your partner an erotic massage with one or two of the essential oils blended with a base oil (see page 189).

- **Seductive scents:** Odour is a sexual magnet, so it's no wonder that many fragrances are linked to the art of allure and seduction. Research shows that pheromones – the natural sexual odours emitted by the body – act as powerful aphrodisiacs. This has lead to some companies mimicking pheromones and bottling them. However, vanilla, sandalwood, ylang-ylang and animal musk (the latter is now synthetically created), have been for centuries – and still are – the key aphrodisiac ingredients of fragrances. Dab one of the following love potions onto such sensual body zones as your décolletage, the tops of your thighs, the nape of your neck and your ankles, and see what happens: Philosophy's Falling in Love, Vivienne Westwood's Boudoir, Aveda's Love, Dior's Hypnotic Poison, Kiehl's Wild Musk, Prescriptives' Flirt and Nari's Karma Sutra Potion.

SEXUAL WORKOUT

Sex is not only one of the richest human experiences,
it can also keep your mind, body and spirit fit, young and beautiful.

BENEFITS OF SEX

The benefits of making love go way beyond merely provoking a contented smile. Psychosexual therapist Judi Keshet-Orr, who teaches sexual-awareness courses, promotes healthy sex as both life-enhancing and beautifying. 'For starters, you feel great', Judi enthuses. 'But sex also keeps you in shape, relaxes you and is a effective de-stresser.'

> There is no greater nor keener pleasure than that of bodily love – and none which is more rational.
>
> Plato (427?–347? BC).

Keep fit with sex

Regular exercise increases your libido, builds sexual stamina and charges your sexual energy. It also boosts the level of DHEA, a hormone that increases sexual excitement. And by being generally fitter, the chances are that you will improve your performance and are more likely to experience earth-shattering orgasms. The act of love-making is a wonderful workout. During sex you can actively firm up zones of your body, in particular your buttocks, thighs and abdominal muscles. As well as toning your body, sex gives you a high similar to the one you get when you've had a good workout session – only a zillion times better. For more powerful orgasms, exercise genital and pelvic muscles by squeezing then holding (repeat several times). Get the most out of sex by making as much noise as you want: this is a great form of release, whether or not you climax.

ENHANCE YOUR SEX LIFE

Unless, like the legendary lover Casanova or the sex guru Anaïs Nin, you have got your bedroom performance down to a fine art, you should be eager to learn more. Experiment: try different positions; be open-minded and discover your hidden passions. Take pleasure in the whole sexual act, be it in intensive foreplay or erotic massage. And do unto your partner what you would like your partner to do unto you.

As a therapist, Judi encourages her clients to develop a better understanding and greater awareness of sex. The magic word that she uses time and time again is 'communication'. This doesn't mean talking dirty, or having a clinical discussion about what you are going to do to each other: it could also be visual or physical communication rather than of the strictly audio variety. We are all aroused in different ways: you might want a soft, romantic caress, whereas your partner might have more animalistic intentions. Try to understand therefore what turns each of you on, and aim to become attuned to your partner's needs.

If your libido is at a low ebb or sex has become as mundane as shaving, a change of scene can revolutionise your sex life: go away for the weekend or try making love somewhere other than the bedroom. You can also better your sex life and send your sexual temperature soaring by indulging in erotica – magazines, videos and lingerie. On a more practical level, Judi suggests the two following books as good 'bed-time' reading: *The Mirror Within*, by Annie Dixon (Quartet, 1985) and *Men & Sex,* by Bernie Zilbergeld (Harper Collins, 1995).

Increase your sexual energy with acupressure

By using finger pressure on a certain point (just above your ankle), health guru Bharti Vyas believes that energy levels can be raised and sexual vitality enhanced. This is Bharti's method: to find the spot, move your finger approximately four finger-widths above the tip of the prominent bone on the inside of the ankle, just behind the shinbone. Measure with one hand and apply pressure with the middle or index finger of the other; maintain the pressure for one minute.

Yoga for sex

Author of *Yoga for Better Sex* (Hamlyn, 1997), yoga guru Vimla Lalvari teaches yoga exercises that work on specific parts of your body, the pelvic-floor stretch being one. Vimla believes that if you do presex yoga, and hold tantric love positions during intercourse, not only will you have a firmer, more toned body, but your sexual experience will be heightened. 'It's preparation work for sex', says Vimla. 'To hold the love positions you need to be supple, flexible and have muscle control. The yoga exercises correspond with certain sexual positions. Practising these with your partner is a form of foreplay, while doing them alone strengthens the parts of your body necessary to hold the poses. The deep breathing you undertake during yoga is also very important to love-making.'

Tantric sex

If the idea of an intensified climax or Vimla's tantalising yogic foreplay appeals to you, then you might want to investigate tantric sex and try Vimla's heart *chakra*, described in further detail below, which creates enormous sexual electricity even before the first physical touch. 'The concept of this Karma Sutra love pose is to transfer energy to each other and attain divine bliss and hours of pleasure', explains Vimla. 'By increasing the build-up of sexual tension before you even touch each other, you heighten arousal and improve love-making.' All these 'no-touching' rules may sound boring, but Vimla assures me that this pose is unbelievably provocative. Give it a try and see how long you can last before leaping on top of each other.

Vimla Lalvari's heart chakra

- Make sure that the room is heated to a comfortable temperature – the only tension present should be sexual tension, not tense muscles because you are shivering with cold.
- Take off all your clothes and sit cross-legged, facing your partner. Sit upright, with your back held straight.
- Hold your hands close to your chest with your palms facing outwards.
- Look each other in the eyes and maintain this gaze throughout (try not to giggle!).
- Simultaneously move your hands slowly down from your chest and outwards towards your partner's hands, then bring them back up until they are level with your chest again, only this time stretch them out further, to the point at which your hands are approximately one inch away from your partner's. Hold this position while gazing into each other's eyes.
- Bring your arms down beside you. Both your mental and physical sexual tension should have increased. Now make love . . .

The erotic massage

An erotic massage not only tones your physique, but also puts you in a state of total relaxation and helps you intuitively to understand and respond to your partner's body. But don't jump in at the deep end: the process should be a long, slow seduction. Ignore the obvious erogenous zones and instead linger on the shoulders, back, armpits, the nape of the neck, scalp, navel, legs and face, and you might just awaken senses that you didn't know existed. During an erotic massage, most recipients experience heightened feelings of arousal, which are often followed by mind-blowing sex. In this unrivalled state of arousal, it is even possible to climax without the assistance of hands-on genital stimulation or intercourse! For your erotic massage to be most effective, invest in a blended aromatherapy oil that includes such aphrodisiac essential oils as sandalwood and ylang-ylang. To experience an erotic nivana, smooth oil that has been pre-warmed over your partner's body and then, using your hands (and if you like also your hair and body), slowly start massaging.

CONTRIBUTORS DIRECTORY

Bobbi Brown
Cosmetics line available at
Harrods in London and Saks
in New York.
UK tel: 0171 730 1234 ex. 277

Sally Brown
Zest Magazine, London.
UK tel: 0171 439 5000

Nicky Clarke, London.
UK tel: 0171 491 4700

Brian Coghlan
The Cranley Clinic, London.
UK tel: 0171 499 3223

Lyndel Costain, Birmingham.
UK tel: 0121 246 6945

Colin Crane
Champneys Health Resort,
Hertfordshire.
UK tel: 01442 291000

Ian Denson
At John Frieda, London and
New York.
UK tel: 0171 636 1401
USA tel: 212 879 1000

Roja Dove
Guerlain, London.
UK tel: 0181 998 9423

Eva Fraser
The Facial Fitness Centre, London.
UK tel: 0171 937 6616

Paula Gilbert
Greyshot Hall Health and Fitness
Resort, Surrey.
UK tel: 01428 604331

Rosie Green
Elle Magazine, London.
UK tel: 0171 437 9011

Mary Greenwell
Agent: Premier, London.
UK tel: 0171 221 2333

Ruby Hammer
Ruby & Millie make-up available at
Harvey Nichols in London.
UK tel: 0171 235 5000

Jo Hansford, London.
UK tel: 0171 495 7774

Susan Harmsworth
E'spa, Surrey.
UK tel: 01252 741 600

Mark Holgate
Vogue Magazine, London.
UK tel: 0171 499 9080

Judi Keshet-Orr
At the Whittington Hospital,
London.
UK tel: 0171 288 3074

Philip Kingsley, London and
New York.
UK tel: 0171 629 4004
USA tel: 212 753 9600

Jeanine Lobell (Stila)
Make-up available at Space NK in
London and Barneys in New York.
UK tel: 0870 607 7060

Eve Lom, London.
UK tel: 0171 935 9988

Vincent Longo, New York.
USA tel: 212 777 0316

Professor Nicholas Lowe
The Cranley Clinic in London and
Santa Monica
UK tel: 0171 499 3223
USA tel: 310 828 8887

Dr Marc Lowenberg
The Marc Lowenberg and Greg
Lituchy Dental Office, New York.
USA tel: 212 586 2890

Jo Malone, London
UK tel: 0171 720 0202
New York: Bergdorf Goodman

Trish McEvoy
Make-up available at Harvey
Nichols in London and Saks
in New York.
UK tel: 0171 235 5000

Sam McKnight
Product range available in the UK
at Boots chemists.

François Nars
Make-up available at Space NK
in London and at Barneys in
New York.
UK tel: 0870 607 7060

Michael O'Connell
Cleansing for change courses,
Somerset.
UK tel: 0145 883 1182

Dr Catherine Orentreich
The Orentreich Medical
Group, LLP, New York.
USA tel: 212 794 0800

Jean Pain
Neuro Linguistic Programming
Teacher, Cambridge.
UK tel: 01223 860356

Radu
Radu's Physical Culture Centre,
New York.
USA tel: 212 581 1995

Dr Robert D. Russell
The Hale Clinic, London.
UK tel: 0171 631 0156
Relaxation CD's available

Bharti Vyas
Bharti Vyas Beauty Clinic,
London.
UK tel: 0171 935 5312
Products available at
Dickens & Jones in London.

PHOTO CREDITS AND ACKNOWLEDGEMENTS

Page 1 by Nick Knight courtesy of © British Vogue/Condé Nast Publications Ltd. Page 2 & 3 Barry Lategan courtesy of © British Vogue/Condé Nast Publications Ltd. Page 4 by and courtesy of © Simon Emmett. Page 7 by Pamela Hanson courtesy of © British Vogue/Condé Nast Publications Ltd. Page 9 & 10 by and courtesy of © Niall McInerney. Page 12 top picture courtesy of © Maybelline New York, bottom picture courtesy of © Revlon. Page 13 top picture courtesy of © Lancôme, bottom picture by Patrick Demarchelier courtesy of © Elizabeth Arden. Page 14 by John Swannell for and courtesy of John Swannell and © Yardley London. Page 15 by E. Sakata for and courtesy of © Lancôme. Page 16 by Santé D'Orazio courtesy of © British Vogue/Condé Nast Publications Ltd. Page 17 by Eugene Aderbari courtesy of © Colourific. Page 18 bottom left by Sipa Press courtesy of © Rex Features Ltd, top right by Charles Sykes courtesy of © Rex Features Ltd. Page 19 middle left courtesy of © Revlon, top right by Brendan Beirne courtesy of © Rex Features Ltd. Pages 20 & 21 by and courtesy of © Andre Dugas. Page 22 by Steichen courtesy of © British Vogue/Condé Nast Publications Ltd. Page 23 top by Arthur Elgort courtesy of © British Vogue/Condé Nast Publications Ltd, bottom by Peter Dackus courtesy of © Robert Harding Syndication. Page 25 by and courtesy of © Niall McInerney. Page 31 by Neil Kirk courtesy of © British Vogue/Condé Nast Publications Ltd. Page 35 by Neil Kirk courtesy of © British Vogue/Condé Nast Publications Ltd. Page 37 by Robin Derrick courtesy of © British Vogue/Condé Nast Publications Ltd. Page 38 by and courtesy of © André Dugas. Page 40 by Andrew Lamb courtesy of © British Vogue/Condé Nast Publications Ltd. Page 41 by and courtesy of © Niall McInerney. Page 43 by John Swannell courtesy of © British Vogue/Condé Nast Publications Ltd. Page 44 by Charles Sykes courtesy of © Rex Features Ltd. Page 47 by Oliver Pearce for 19 courtesy of © Robert Harding Syndication. Page 53 by Neil Kirk courtesy of © British Vogue/Condé Nast Publications Ltd. Page 55 by Piero Gemelli courtesy of © Tatler/Condé Nast Publications Ltd. Pages 56 & 57 by Ian Skelton courtesy of © Tatler/Condé Nast Publications Ltd. Page 60 by David Oldfield for 19 courtesy of © Robert Harding Syndication. Page 63 by and courtesy of © Niall McInerney. Page 65 by Arthur Elgort courtesy of © British Vogue/Condé Nast Publications Ltd. Page 66 courtesy of © Rex Features Ltd. Page 69 by Neil Kirk courtesy of © British Vogue/Condé Nast Publications Ltd. Page 70 by Richard Young courtesy of © Rex Features Ltd. Page 71 bottom of Jo Levin by Andrew Douglas courtesy of © Andrew Douglas and Jo Levin, top by K. Wisniewski courtesy of © Rex Features Ltd. Pages 72 & 73 by Arthur Elgort courtesy of © British Vogue/Condé Nast Publications Ltd. Pages 74, 77 and 81 by and courtesy of © Andre Dugas. Page 79 by and courtesy of © Niall McInerney. Pages 82 & 83 by Paul Cox for Nicky Clarke courtesy of © Nicky Clarke/Modus PR. Page 85 by Keith Henderson for Marie Claire courtesy of © Robert Harding Syndication. Pages 86 & 87 by and courtesy of © André Dugas. Page 89 by and courtesy of © Niall McInerney. Page 91 by Sean Cunningham courtesy of © British Vogue/Condé Nast Publications Ltd. .Pages 94 & 95 by and courtesy of © Niall McInerney. Page 97 by Regan Cameron courtesy of © British Vogue/Condé Nast Publications Ltd. Page 99 by David Parfitt courtesy of © British Vogue/Condé Nast Publications Ltd. Page 101 courtesy of © Caci International. Page 105 by Robert Erdmann courtesy of © British Vogue/Condé Nast Publications Ltd. Page 106 by Andre Dugas courtesy of Eva Fraser. Page 109 by Hiromasa for Marie Claire courtesy of © Robert Harding Syndication. Pages 110 & 111 by Jorgen Ahlstrom courtesy of © Tatler/Condé Nast Publications Ltd. Page 114 by and courtesy of © Niall McInerney. Page 115 by Graeme Montgomery courtesy of © Tatler/Condé Nast Publications Ltd. Page 117 by Robin Derrick courtesy of © British Vogue/Condé Nast Publications Ltd. Page 119 by and courtesy of © André Dugas. Page 123 by Clive Arrowsmith courtesy of © British Vogue/Condé Nast Publications Ltd. Pages 126 & 127 by Pamela Hanson courtesy of © British Vogue/Condé Nast Publications Ltd. Page 128 by Arthur Elgort courtesy of © British Vogue/Condé Nast Publications Ltd. Pages 130 & 131 by and courtesy of © Andre Dugas. Page 133 by Jorgen Ahlstrom courtesy of © Tatler/Condé Nast Publications Ltd. Page 135 by Robin Derrick courtesy of © British Vogue/Condé Nast Publications Ltd. Page 141 by Hans Feurer courtesy of © Tatler/Condé Nast Publications Ltd. Page 143 of Radu courtesy of Radu Physical Culture. Page 144 by Robert Erdmann courtesy of © British Vogue/Condé Nast Publications Ltd. Page 147 by Wendy Carrig for 19 courtesy of © Robert Harding Syndication. Page 149 Arthur Elgort courtesy of © British Vogue/Condé Nast Publications Ltd. Page 151 by Simon Bottomley for Options courtesy of © Robert Harding Syndication. Page 153 by and courtesy of © André Dugas. Page 155 by Mark Mattock courtesy of © British Vogue/Condé Nast Publications Ltd. Pages 156 & 157 by Piero Gemelli courtesy of © Tatler/Condé Nast Publications Ltd. Page 158 by Graeme Montgomery for Options courtesy of © Robert Harding Syndication. Page 160 & 165 by and courtesy of © André Dugas. Page 163 by Tim Walker courtesy of © British Vogue/Condé Nast Publications Ltd. Page 169 by Robert Erdmann courtesy of © British Vogue/Condé Nast Publications Ltd. Page 173 courtesy of © Champneys Health Resort. Page 174 both pictures of Chiva-Som Health Resort courtesy of Becall Harris Associates, London. Page 175 top courtesy of © Meiv Griffins Resort Hotel & Givenchy Spa, bottom Chiva-Som Health Resort courtesy of Becall Harris Associates, London. Pages 176 & 177 courtesy of © Greyshot Hall Health & Fitness Retreat. Page 179 by Brian Nice courtesy of © Cosmopolitan/National Magazines. Page 180 by Leis for Freundin courtesy of © Robert Harding Syndication. Page 182 by L. Donato for Freudin courtesy of © Robert Harding Syndication. Page 184 courtesy of © Elfried Blaes and Clinique La Prairie, Clarets, Montreux, Switzerland. Page 185 courtesy of © Champneys Health Resort. Page 186 by Lisa Linda courtesy of © Company/National Magazines.

First published in Great Britain in 1999 by Weidenfeld & Nicolson

A CIP catalogue record for this book is available from the British Library
ISBN 0 297 824295

Picture research: Sandra Morris
Designed by: Peter Butler
Set in: Akzidenz Grotesk

Printed in Italy by Printer Trento srl

Weidenfeld & Nicolson
The Orion Publishing Group Ltd
5 Upper Saint Martin's Lane
London WC2H 9EA

DISCLAIMER

The suggestions in this book are not intended as a substitute for professional medical advice and any application of the contents of *The Beauty Manual* is at the reader's sole discretion and risk. The publishers, author and contributors are, therefore, not responsible for any injuries, allergies or other problems whatsoever arising from beauty treatments, products, information or advice given in this book.

CORRECTIONS

Every effort has been made to ensure that the credits, information, product names and directory are accurate. However, if any errors are brought to the attention of the publishers, they will be more than happy to make any corrections in the event of a reprint.

ACKNOWLEDGEMENTS

The author would like to thank everyone who helped with the book. In particular, she would like to say a special thank you to the following people who gave their time, information, quotes, tips and expert advice: Rosie Green, Jean Pain, Bharti Vyas, Ruby Hammer, Bobbi Brown, Mark Holgate, Mary Greenwell, Trish McEvoy, Jeanine Lobell, Vincent Longo, François Nars, Nicky Clarke, Andrew Clark, Philip Kingsley, Jo Hansford, Ian Denton, John Frieda, Sam McKnight, Dr Catherine Orentreich, Professor Nicholas Lowe, Eva Fraser, Dr Marc Lowenberg, Jo Malone, Eve Lom, The Untouchables, Mr Brian Coghlan, Radu, Sally Brown, Michael O'Connell, Susan Harmsworth, Roja Dove, Dr Robert D. Russell, Colin Crane, Paula Gilbert, Lyndel Costain, Judi Keshet-Orr, Vimla Lalvari, Orlando Pita, Deepak Chopra, Kevin Mancuso, Frédéric Fekkai, Oribe, John Frieda, Marcia Kilgore, Charles Worthington, Dick Page, Millie Kendall, Maggie Hunt, Jo Levin, Louis Licari, Antoinette Beenders, Gronya Logan, Christine Ambrose, Cristina Carlino, Polly Mellen, William P. Lauder.

The author would also like to thank the model agents and PR's who made interviews, tips and quotes possible including: Elaine Dugas and Jonathan Phang at IMG Models; Miranda Denoff at Elite Premier; Paula Karaiskos and Gavin Boardman at Storm Models; Jane Wood at Models 1; Jez Felwick at Panic; Caroline Kannreuther at Lancôme; Elise at Jason Weidenberg; Valerie Oula at Ford Models; Marian Scott at Revlon; Humaira Sadiq at Procter & Gamble; Dee Carpenter at Dee Carpenter PR; Julia Brignall at Linda Land PR; Tim Howard at Art & Commerce; Chris O'Leary at Jed Root; Owen Walker and Tashia Hudson at Dowelwalker; Isabelle Remanda-Harpham and Mina Kuhera at MKPR; Emma Elliot and Julie Winkler at Modus PR; Sandra Boland at L'oreal and Maybelline; Julian Sheldon at TCS; Michelle Seabrook at Cellex-C; Jenni Patterson at Wizard PR; Jane McCorriston at Elizabeth Arden; Clare Ripper at Clinique; Louise Dorey at Shiseido; James de Lacey at Kanebo; Renee Dunn at The Chopra Centre; Hannah Boulton at Harvey Nichols; Emma Wilson at Guerlain; Jane Seymour at Clarins; Natalie Holloway at Prescriptives; Gene Rodda at Radu's; Christina Thomas at Champneys; Erica Frei, Anna MacLellan at A.N.A; Jeff Becall at Becall Harris; David Lurie at Givenchy Spa.

Sandra would like to say a very big thank you to her project manager Claire Colreavy, and also to Susan Haynes and Michael Dover at Weidenfeld & Nicolson and her agent Fiona Batty at Peter, Fraser & Dunlop for giving her the opportunity to write and produce this challenging book. Sandra wishes to dedicate *The Beauty Manual* to her husband Bart.